LIVING WELL WITH ASTHMA

ఖ LIVING WELL WITH ASTHMA

Michael R. Freedman, Ph.D.
Samuel J. Rosenberg, Ph.D.
Cynthia L. Divino, Ph.D.

THE GUILFORD PRESS
New York   London

© 1998 The Guilford Press
A Division of Guilford Publications, Inc.
72 Spring Street, New York, NY 10012
http://www.guilford.com

The information in this volume is not intended as a substitution for consultation with health care professionals. Each individual's health concerns should be evaluated by a qualified professional.

Printed in the United States of America

This book is printed on acid-free paper.

Last digit is print number: 9 8 7 6 5 4 3 2 1

Library of Congress Cataloging-in-Publication Data

Freedman, Michael R.
    Living with asthma / Michael R. Freedman, Samuel J. Rosenberg, Cynthia L. Divino
        p.   cm.
    Includes bibliographical references and index.
    ISBN 1-57230-318-2 (hardcover: alk. paper). — ISBN 1-57230-051-5 (pbk.: alk. paper)
    1. Asthma—Psychological aspects. 2. Asthma—Social aspects.
I. Rosenberg, Samuel J. II. Divino, Cynthia L. III. Title.
RC591.F74 1998
616.2'38—DC21   97-48747
                                                                    CIP

To my family, especially Elizabeth,
Aaron, Sarah, and Emma

MRF

To my family, with special thanks to Patti
and my Mom for their perserverance

SJR

To Daniel, for everything you have given me,
and to my parents, Dominick and Angie Divino,
for a lifetime of love and support

CLD

and for our patients

✎ CONTENTS

Part IV. Living Well in the Wider World

Appendix

Index

♨ Foreword

Asthma and other chronic illnesses create intense and unique stresses on patients, families, and physicians, raising issues that must be addressed both inside and outside the medical setting. While asthma's overt signs and symptoms are all too familiar to sufferers—continuously or intermittently disrupting normal functioning and occasionally creating a life-threatening emergency—its subtler impact on everyday life, even when the disease is under apparent control, is often less well understood. Synthesizing knowledge gained from years of working with asthma patients and their families, Michael Freedman, Samuel Rosenberg, and Cynthia Divino shed light on vital personal and social issues in this invaluable resource.

Psychological distress caused by asthma can substantially affect self-image, family and community interactions, and compliance with medical care, and can even lead to the initiation or propagation of symptoms. The complex interplay of psychological and physical well-being is clearly illuminated in this book, in whose numerous illustrations and examples all readers will recognize aspects of their own experience. Patients and their families will also gain insight into the ways they may be allowing asthma to constrain their lives unnecessarily, and will learn the skills they need to increase their comfort level within relationships, in social settings, and in the workplace.

Ideal for patients, their family members, and significant others, this book should also be required reading for health care providers. Without an understanding of the psychosocial aspects of asthma, optimal medical treatment is hindered. More frequent and higher doses of drugs are required when the psychosocial and environmental triggers are not addressed, and little is accomplished by developing effective new pharmaceutical agents if stress causes patients not to use medications as prescribed.

I applaud the efforts of Drs. Freedman, Rosenberg, and Divino to draw from their unique clinical experiences to focus on the treatment of whole patients and their social environments. Helping patients reduce the adverse psychosocial effects of asthma will be as effective as any current or future medication in enabling them to truly live well.

JAMES D. CRAPO, MD
Chairman, Department of Medicine
Executive Vice President for Academic Affairs
National Jewish Medical and Research Center
Denver, Colorado

Introduction

When you have asthma, you need more than physical care to help you breathe easily. The disease may reside in your lungs, but your entire life can be affected by the illness. Medication may open your airways, but how has the need for it altered your self-image and consequently your relationships? Avoidance of asthma triggers may keep you from wheezing, but what has a modified lifestyle done to your social life?

If your asthma treatment does not address the emotional and social aspects of the disease, you may find your physical symptoms out of control as well. You'll certainly find that your life isn't as full or as fulfilling as you'd like it to be.

In our work with asthma patients at the National Jewish Medical and Research Center, we were struck by the inescapable impact of psychosocial issues in every facet of asthma management. Patients come to the National Jewish Center in Denver, world renowned in the treatment of lung, allergic, and immune diseases, from all over the country, typically because their asthma is under poor control. Some of the asthma patients we saw were reluctant to follow medical advice because they were afraid that their treatment regimen would harm or restrict their job, their relationships, or their lifestyle. Others followed their doctors' recommendations, but adjusting to the disease was taking a major toll on their emotional, social, or occupational

1

functioning. Obviously something was missing from the care and self-care these people were getting.

The health care professionals at National Jewish determined that what was needed in virtually every case was *treatment of the asthma patient as a whole person*. Successful adaptation to this chronic, cyclical, sometimes unpredictable disease demands attention to emotional, mental, and social difficulties as well as respiratory problems. "I'm not just a pair of lungs!" cried one of our patients, succinctly summing up the emotional anguish that can result when we try to treat any disease by isolating body from mind and spirit.

The solution is the biopsychosocial management of asthma. In a relatively rare approach, National Jewish integrates cutting-edge advances in medical care with psychosocial treatment that uncovers and addresses problems in productivity, family, functioning, or happiness stemming from the diagnosis of asthma or the treatment regimen already in place. Physicians work with psychologists, psychiatrists, and social workers to arrive at a final treatment plan by examining the whole person, not just the disease. The psychosocial staff also works with physicians to modify treatment, where necessary, to increase the likelihood that medical recommendations will be followed.

After twenty-eight years of combined experience in treating patients with asthma at National Jewish and subsequently in private practice, we can say with confidence that the biopsychosocial approach to treating asthma is a success. Clearing away psychological and social obstacles to treatment compliance improves asthma. Adapting to the illness emotionally and mentally as well as physically leads to a happier, healthier lifestyle.

We wrote this book because we want you, like our patients, to live well with asthma. If you take medication only rarely, with only an occasional asthma flare-up, you're likely to cruise through life with only minor modifications to your lifestyle. But if your asthma is moderate to severe—now or at any point in the cycle of asthma or the stages of life—adjustment to the disease may not come so easily. *Don't give up on leading the kind of life you want.* You don't need to resign yourself to an existence ruled by a pair of faulty lungs. You don't have to settle for breathing fairly easily but living pretty poorly.

This book is intended to guide you past the pitfalls of adapting to asthma through information and inspiration. Based on our experience, we'll describe the emotional and social factors that usually arise with asthma so you can anticipate them and adjust to them without sacrificing what's important to you in life. We'll give you some proven techniques for building a foundation of self-knowledge that will serve you over a lifetime of change and growth. In every chapter, we'll present case examples—some real people with identifying information altered and disguised to protect their confidentiality, some composites, all drawn from a rich variety of clinical experience—to illustrate how others have met the challenges you may be facing, now or in the future.

These examples should help you understand that you're not alone, grappling with this illness in a vacuum. The National Center for Health Statistics reports that the incidence of asthma in 1994 (the last year the survey was conducted) was *14,562,000* cases, with the incidence of asthma increasing forty-six percent between 1982 and 1993. Those figures, too, compelled us to write this book. Despite the fact that asthma is indisputably on the rise, and that numerous books on its medical management (including some reflecting recent trends toward alternative medicine such as herbal and homeopathic techniques) are available, precious little information has been disseminated on living well with asthma through psychosocial adaptation. We hope this book closes that gap.

We do not offer any medical advice in this book, and in no sense is this book meant to substitute for a physician's advice and care. For answers to any medical question about asthma, always consult your doctor. And please make use of the many other resources available to you—including those listed in the Appendix—for more information on medical and other aspects of asthma. Thanks to the research commitment of medical centers like National Jewish, advances in medical care are being made at a rapid rate today, and we know you'll want to stay abreast of those and other developments.

In the meantime, we fervently hope that your physician will cooperate enthusiastically with your efforts to take a biopsychosocial approach to self-care and will support those efforts with a like-minded approach of his or her own. It's no exaggeration to say that patient–physician teamwork, when it's directed at body, mind, and spirit, can lead not only to a better life *with* asthma but also to a better life *than before* asthma. What you gain from a successful adaptation to this disease will serve you well in all areas of your life.

HOW TO USE THIS BOOK

This book is meant for those newly diagnosed with asthma as well as those experiencing a worsening of symptoms at any point in life. Ideally, it will help you solve problems you're currently facing and anticipate others. Because your relationships with others are an integral part of your adaptation to asthma, you might want to share the book with the important people in your life. Use it as a self-help guide, but don't hesitate to seek professional assistance when you need it. Throughout the following chapters, we'll point out circumstances that may call for a helping hand.

Parts I and II explain what asthma is biologically and how it is likely to affect you psychologically and socially. These chapters give you a base of knowledge about emotional and social adaptation to asthma and set you on the road to self-knowledge about your unique life with asthma by offering tools and techniques to help you adapt following diagnosis and at various stages in your life.

- Chapter 1 describes the biopsychosocial model that we use to understand and resolve problems created by asthma, supplies a biological overview of the disease, defines asthma-related terms, and dispels common myths about asthma.
- The diagnosis of asthma and your management of the disease over time may change your body image. Chapter

2 explains how to recognize such changes in perception and what to do about them.

- Chapter 3 describes asthma's common effects on your feelings and gives you methods for examining beliefs that may be causing you unnecessary emotional pain.
- Chapter 4 describes how faulty beliefs and perceptions may interfere with your medical management and how you can prevent this from hindering your health and happiness.
- Chapter 5 helps you understand how your response to the diagnosis of asthma can hamper your adaptation to the illness. Understanding the typical diagnosis–response–adaptation process and your particular responses to difficult or stressful situations will give you the insight you need to move forward into living better with asthma.

Parts III and IV are devoted to specific situations in different areas of your life. Here is information on the all-important adaptation of your family, including suggestions for keeping your marriage sound, maintaining a satisfactory parental role, and managing life when your child has asthma too. Life exists beyond the doors of home, of course, so we offer chapters on adapting to asthma at work and in your social life as well. Finally, recommendations for keeping the all-important doctor–patient relationship thriving are provided.

- You're not the only one who receives the diagnosis of asthma; your family gets it along with you. Nor are you the only one who must adapt. Chapter 6 acknowledges that, without family adaptation, your individual adaptation will suffer. Here are tips for using flexibility, communication, and other resources to adapt collectively as well as individually. *These methods form the foundation for successful adaptation within any group setting.* In the family, they enable you to switch roles, address the needs of your children at various ages, and facilitate proactive problem solving.

- Chapter 7 deals candidly with the often-evaded subject of asthma's effect on sexuality. Included here are suggestions for keeping your head from interfering in your sex life and practical tips for the physical act of lovemaking.
- Genetically, your children are somewhat predisposed to having asthma. Chapter 8 will help you raise a well-adjusted asthmatic child, in the process shedding some light on how your upbringing may be causing problems in your own adaptation right now.
- Turning to the outside world, Chapter 9 discusses an all-too-familiar problem: poorly managed asthma due to attempts to hide the disease at work. Case examples and employer testimonials will show you that fears about the perceptions of employers and coworkers are usually unfounded. We'll show you how to make flexibility and communication work for everyone at the workplace.
- The same rules of thumb that keep your family functioning can help you maintain a stimulating social life despite your respiratory problems. Chapter 10 gives details.
- Are you getting all you should from your relationship with your doctor? Chapter 11 enumerates ways to examine your own perceptions and put yourself in your physician's shoes so that the two of you can reach an understanding on the best approach to keeping you healthy and happy.

No single book can possibly answer all your questions, so we hope you'll investigate some of the other resources listed in our Appendix. Adaptation—to asthma or any other element in your life—is an ongoing process, and the best way to meet new challenges with alacrity is to stay informed.

In the meantime, we hope this book will help you breathe easier. As an asthmatic person, you know better than anyone why *breathing easier* has become a metaphor for much more than inhaling and exhaling freely. It means feeling relaxed and confident, vital and prepared for whatever you face. It means living well with asthma, and that's what we wish for you.

PART I

YOU ARE NOT ALONE . . .

❧ Chapter 1

"Asthma: It's Just a Breathing Problem, Right?"

For years, John had enjoyed spending the weekend working around the house. He cut the grass, trimmed the bushes, and mended the broken gutters. He found this outdoor work a pleasurable change from his weekdays of laboring with pen and paper as an architect. His childhood asthma, long forgotten, had returned, however, and now John was finding this yardwork increasingly difficult.

John was also becoming angry and short-tempered. He snapped at his wife, Mary, over the slightest conflict, and since he was home more often, he and Mary were arguing more and more frequently.

"I don't know what's happening to me," John lamented in our office. "I can't push that lawn mower around because I get too tired. And the dust, grass, and pollen seem to make my chest even tighter. So now I spend my weekends inside, watching television. I'm getting fed up with sitting in a recliner most of the day, but there's really nothing else I can do."

"Now, John," Mary retorted, "you're just taking care of yourself. I don't mind doing some of the yardwork if it helps you."

"And that's something else," John said angrily. "Mary shouldn't be doing that stuff around the house. That's a man's job."

THE IMPACT OF ASTHMA

The return of John's asthma was diagnosed accurately by his physician, and the medical treatment prescribed is appropriate for his particular condition. Yet John is not feeling well, not doing well at home or at work, not living well. *Why not?*

Because medical treatment alone is not enough—not for John and probably not for you. Asthma does not affect just the lungs; it is an illness that touches all aspects of life. Obviously, difficulty breathing can pose various physical challenges, as John discovered. But it can also drastically change how you feel about yourself, your family, your work, and more. John is beginning to feel sad and helpless because he has lost not only a satisfying activity that was part of his weekly routine but also a valued role in his family. This shift in family roles—letting his wife do a "man's job"—makes John believe he is less of a man.

Does it have to be that way? Is there, as he currently believes, nothing else John can do?

Absolutely not. For John and for all of us, living well with asthma begins with awareness that asthma can create problems beyond those surrounding the need to control the physical illness. Address these social and psychological difficulties along with the physical symptoms and you stand an excellent chance of living better with this disease.

It shouldn't come as a surprise that asthma can have far-reaching effects. We've all experienced how even a brief illness can impact ourselves and others. For example, children quickly learn the positive and negative effects of an illness such as chicken pox. On the positive side, they need not go to school or do homework, they are fed their favorite foods, and they receive constant attention from parents. On the negative side, they don't feel particularly good because of the chicken pox, and they cannot spend time playing with friends. These lessons are learned so well that, later, children sometimes use a physical complaint such as "My throat hurts," to try to avoid school. So we discover early that an illness can have both psychological and social consequences.

While as children we grasp the interpersonal effects of an illness, it's not until later that most of us realize psychological and social events can affect our body and how it works. Probably one of the most widely accepted ideas is that psychological stress can predispose us to physical problems, such as peptic ulcers or tension headaches. The corporate executive whose fast-paced and stress-filled life requires him to keep a bottle of antacid in his bottom desk drawer and a roll of antacids in his coat pocket is a familiar picture. Similarly, some people note that strong emotions, such as anger, can prompt an asthma attack. Once they're short of breath, fear and panic can make breathing even worse. These observations suggest that the relationship between the body and psychological or social concerns is bidirectional; it is a two-way street. Just as being ill can affect how you feel, think, and relate to others, your emotions, thoughts, and relationships can influence how your body works. A wealth of research indicates that if John remains angry and helpless about the limitations asthma has imposed on his body, there's a good chance he will begin to lose physical control of the disease as well.

THE BIOPSYCHOSOCIAL APPROACH TO ASTHMA

This bidirectional approach to understanding physical illness is called the *biopsychosocial model*. The prefix *bio* refers to the biological aspects of a disease, such as the muscle spasms, inflammation, and mucous secretions during an asthma attack. John, for one, noted that the dust and grass in his yard seemed to worsen his asthma. *Psycho* refers to both the psychological effects of a disease on a patient and the role of psychological factors in precipitating or maintaining the disease. Within the psychological realm, John was feeling sad and angry because he could no longer do the yardwork. Finally, *social* alludes to the role of interpersonal issues in a disease, like Mary's decision to do the yardwork because of John's asthma. According to the biopsychosocial model, all three elements are equal partners in creating or maintaining an illness. This means that to understand the illness, you need to look simultaneously at all three—body, mind, and interpersonal relationships—and that you cannot view one as primary and the others as secondary.

The biopsychosocial model contrasts sharply with the approach taught traditionally in medical schools. The traditional approach is based on what is called the *biomedical model* because it dismisses the psychosocial aspects of illness and focuses solely on biological factors. Not only are the patient's and family's responses to the illness disregarded, but also physical causes are considered the sole sources of disease. The biomedical model assumes that there are no important relationships between the mind and the body, that everything to be learned about an illness can be discovered through an understanding of how the body works. This approach, in its extreme form, is partly responsible for the growing specialization of medicine. If the body is separated from the mind, the logical extreme tells us the body can be divided into separate organ systems that can be understood almost independently from one another. Thus, a patient goes to a cardiologist for heart problems, a nephrologist for kidney difficulties, or maybe a pulmonologist for lung concerns. And if you have many symptoms, you find yourself going to many doctors. Who, then, is responsible for coordinating treatment? Who makes sure that the doctors talk to one another? You are. Although it is important for you to learn about your illnesses, it is not necessarily desirable for you to be the person making sure that all the doctors know what the others are doing. And that is one serious consequence of the biomedical model—specialists are interested in organ systems, not the patient.

The philosophical difference between these two models is important to you as a patient because it comes into the doctor's office along with you and your physician. Within the biomedical model, emotional reactions to illness frequently remain undetected or ignored by the physician because they are not seen as relevant to treating the patient. In contrast, many patients want to talk about what it is like to live with asthma yet believe that their physicians lack either the time or the interest. As a result, patients are left feeling either sad, angry, or frustrated with their physicians. Over and over, we've seen that when doctor and patient hold different ideas about disease, conflicts inevitably arise. Beth describes one conflict quite well:

&ewm; "My doctor just won't listen to me. She just comes in, asks me to take some deep breaths, listens to my chest, and either increases or decreases my steroids [a drug often prescribed for severe asthma, as you may already know]. She then asks me how I'm doing, but it almost seems like she's walking out the door while she's asking. It's so frustrating, but she's pretty busy, and I know there's another patient waiting."

Recent psychological research confirms that we all want the interpersonal qualities in our doctors that Beth misses in hers. According to several studies, patients desire primarily two things from their doctors: the technical ability to treat their physical problems and the capacity to create an atmosphere of trust and confidence. The first requirement is generally satisfied when you leave your appointment with both a diagnosis and a treatment plan that will eventually make you feel better. To supply the second, the physician must listen to your difficulties, even if they fall within the psychological or social areas, convey feelings of caring and sensitivity about the problems, and be both friendly and warm during the meeting. Interestingly, these interpersonal qualities seem to be much more important in satisfaction with physicians than patients' perception of doctors' competence. Therefore, the biomedical model, which empha-sizes technical expertise, is bound to fall short. Patients are simply happier with physicians who are both technically knowl-edgeable about and sensitive to the psychological and social consequences of illness.

This research, of course, describes the expectations of the average patient, and you are not average. You have your own ideas about your illness and your doctor. Perhaps you don't want to believe that asthma affects other parts of your life. Maybe you want your doctor to simply fix you so your lungs will work well again. If you firmly believed that asthma is all about chest tightness, wheezing, and gulping for air, you wouldn't be reading this sentence. Why? Because you would never have picked up a book about living well with asthma. The mere fact that you are reading this book suggests you know there is more to your asthma than just a list of symptoms. You already believe parts of the biopsychosocial model, even though you may never have heard about it before.

UNDERSTANDING *YOUR* ASTHMA

So, what does this model mean for you? Obviously, your illness should be considered more than just a specific bodily problem. A wide range of nonbiological factors are involved in the making of an illness, and all must be taken into account in treating and managing the illness. Psychological factors include how you view past illnesses and physicians, how you cope with stress, and your personality style. Social influences might include your parents' or other family members' experiences with similar illness, family reactions to your illness, and religious or cultural influences. Because each of us brings a different set of these factors to the bodily problem, the meaning of the illness and the experience of it are unique for each person.

Illness is thus a subjective experience, dependent on your unique perspective. This means that two people can have identical symptoms and diseases yet experience and perceive their illness differently and react differently to it as well. For example, two men of similar age are diagnosed with asthma. Unfortunately, one man's father also suffered from asthma and died suddenly from an asthma attack. This patient reacted to the diagnosis with dread and anxiety. He felt as if he had been handed a death sentence. In contrast, the other man took the diagnosis calmly and began to read about his disease, hoping to learn more about it. The difference between these two men was not the disease but rather the psychological factors they brought to that disease. This difference in turn influenced their perception of the disease and their reaction to it. We all have a unique wealth of experience that eventually becomes intertwined with asthma. These experiences help shape our view of and reaction to asthma.

This is not meant to dismiss the importance of illness severity or the specific symptoms in the development of the experience of asthma, but rather to highlight that there are other, nonphysical factors involved in that process that are just as influential.

Understanding and addressing these other factors can help you live better with asthma. Knowing that there are many different circumstances shaping your illness and that your case is unique will support all your ongoing efforts, and you will carry this understanding with you for a lifetime. But you will not have a full understanding of your own asthma unless you understand the general nature of the disease as well as the many factors in your particular case. Let's start by clearing away a few persistent myths about the disease.

For reasons that we'll be exploring throughout this book, living with asthma creates high levels of various emotions that beg to be controlled. It's only natural that patients and families sometimes seek comfort in fallacies that assuage their anger and fear, fulfill their hopes, or affirm their protective love—no matter how briefly. Unfortunately, whether you're clinging to myths yourself or having them foisted on you by friends and family, in the long run they can only stand in the way of your living better with asthma.

MISCONCEPTIONS ABOUT ASTHMA

Myth #1: It's all in your head, right?

Asthma is not entirely in your head any more than it is only physical. No matter how much stress, turmoil, conflict, or trauma exists in your life, you would not have developed asthma without the underlying respiratory disease. While asthma is not psychosomatic (created by the mind), psychological or social influences do affect the disease, as we've already said. For example, it is accepted that stress and certain strong feelings can trigger an asthma attack in some individuals. And, once you're short of breath, panic or anxiety can worsen the symptoms. In our view, you need to consider biological, psychological, and social factors all at the same time. So, while asthma is not all in your head, it's also not all in your lungs.

Unfortunately, the belief that asthma is all in your head is probably the most common misconception about the disease, and you'll undoubtedly encounter it more than once. Best to be prepared. Keep in mind that someone who says your asthma is all in your head may be communicating any of a wide range of thoughts and feelings:

• One possibility is that the person is not knowledgeable about asthma and truly believes that it is an illness of the mind. If a lack of information seems probable, you might use the comment as an opportunity to educate the person about asthma. Breathing is such an automatic function that few people think about their lungs until something is wrong with them.

• Could the person who says it's all in your head be expressing the wish that you will get better? Others who care about you may believe that if you try harder to breathe better, your asthma symptoms will diminish. In this case the person feels helpless to do anything to help you and wants to give you encouragement. Unfortunately, because asthma is not entirely in your head, at times you also may feel helpless to control the symptoms. Not only that, you may find yourself annoyed with this person who seems, however unintentionally, to be blaming you for your symptoms. After all, this person is telling you that you should be able to consciously control your symptoms, sometimes only with more willpower. As you probably know, that can annoy someone who is having trouble breathing.

• Physicians are not immune to this myth. Your physician might suggest that the asthma is psychosomatic when months have passed and, despite all the doctor's work, your symptoms persist. What likely occurs during these moments is that the physician is feeling both helpless and frustrated, and therefore succumbs to the urge to shift responsibility to you. Understandably, this shift in blame can leave you feeling angry, frustrated, and demoralized. In this case some people seek a new physician (see Chapter 11), but others do nothing, remaining depressed and guilt-ridden. If you find yourself in this position, before changing doctors you might try to discuss the frustration and helplessness you share with your physician and then develop a new treatment plan with him or her, possibly including a second opinion. Of course, this is not an easy task. But blaming one another for the problems only serves to alienate you from each other.

This kind of blaming can take more subtle forms than just a blunt "It's all in your head." For example:

․ George returns home from work one night to find his wife Jessica short of breath. They had planned to go out for dinner with someone from his office, but now the plan appears in jeopardy. George says angrily, "Why do you always have an asthma attack before our dinner engagements?" implying Jessica's asthma is deliberate and controllable. Jessica replies, "But George, you know I've been fighting a cold all week. Now it's got the better of me. I'm sorry we can't go to dinner tonight. I know it's frustrating for you, but it's also frustrating for me."

Although we don't know whether, in fact, Jessica used her illness to avoid the dinner engagement, the case illustrates how suggestions that asthma is controllable with more willpower, more effort, or a better attitude can serve to blame you, the patient, for your illness.

Myth #2: "Asthma isn't serious. I mean, no one dies from asthma."

Depending on how you define asthma, between seven and twenty million people in the United States have it, two to five million of whom are children. In fact, recent epidemiological research suggests that asthma is becoming more prevalent and more severe. About five thousand people in the United States die from asthma each year. A recent study suggested that the same number have asthma listed on the death certificate but not as the immediate cause of death. In addition, death rates from asthma are rising, especially among the elderly and children. Asthma is the leading cause of school absenteeism and pediatric admissions to hospitals. Americans spend about $3 billion every year on asthma medication and an additional $2 billion on doctor visits and hospitalizations.

The cover of the May 26, 1997, issue of *Newsweek* was plastered with the huge headline "The Scary Spread of Asthma and How to Protect Your Kids"—just one example of how the prevalence of asthma is being brought more and more to the public's attention today. Still, it will probably take some time before conventional wisdom thoroughly adopts a serious attitude toward the disease. That's because minimizing its seriousness answers a strong emotional need.

Most people need to deny the dangerousness of the illness, because they would otherwise find themselves overwhelmed by distressing feelings. Anxiety, sadness, rage, and vulnerability can all be minimized by downplaying the significance of asthma. Both you and your family and friends may feel happier viewing asthma as a small problem that is easily controlled rather than as a chronic, and possibly lethal, illness requiring attention.

Fortunately, there is a safer middle ground between abject fear and ignorant bliss. It's called knowledge. Learn more about the disease, understand and comply with your medical treatment, and do all you can to discern the impact of personal psychological and social factors on the disease. You don't have to go it alone. Health care professionals view asthma seriously, and they can help you do so too. Make it clear that you expect to be kept informed. Knowledge is not only your most reliable armor against fear, but it also can help you convince those around you to take your disease seriously too.

Myth #3: "There's a cure for asthma, right?"

There is no cure for asthma. Asthma can be controlled or managed, it may come and go, but it cannot be cured. However, for most people the wish for a cure persists. Some people ask directly for a "magic pill," others search the newsstands for a new discovery, and still others pressure their physicians to prescribe a yet-to-be-tried medication. The important people in your life may look for a cure as well. By doing so, they may place unnecessary pressure on you to spend time searching for a cure rather than managing your illness. *The cure for asthma is management; the cure for people who believe there is a cure is education.*

We all wish for a cure for asthma. And most of our personal experiences with medical illnesses support that wish. We feel sick, we get a diagnosis and a medication, and eventually we feel better. That is the course of most medical conditions, from a common cold to a broken leg. Most of us are less comfortable and familiar with illnesses that are chronic and require management, without immediate hope for a cure. We don't want to suggest that you give up hope. Just don't let your hope interfere with management of your asthma.

Myth #4: "It's your mother's fault that you have asthma."

Somewhere, sometime, someone is going to tell you that your mother is probably to blame for your asthma. Why? Because, for decades, mental health professionals examined the mother-child relationship, trying to figure out how it influences both the development and the course of asthma. Some elegant theories based on these observations were developed, but their accuracy is now suspect, and all that remains is the myth of blaming your mother. Nonetheless, it's helpful to review several of these theories in case you need to protect and defend your mother from such accusations.

One theory stated that asthma develops when the mother has mixed feelings about having a child. Concretely, this uncertainty can be seen in mothers who alternate between smothering their children with hugs and pushing them away. The child, in turn, senses the mother's mixed feelings and feels angry and hurt. But the child believes that Mother would strictly punish him or her if the child directly expressed these feelings. To resolve this conflict, the child develops asthma. The asthma attack is thus seen as communicating three feelings. First, it reflects anxiety about being separated from the mother.

Second, it is a suppressed cry for help to the mother, a hope that she will stay and protect the child. Finally, it is an indirect expression of rage toward the mother for being ambivalent, for not loving the child unconditionally. While an elegant theory, research has not borne out the idea that mothers are to blame for their children's asthma because of their mixed feelings toward the children.

Other studies of the influence of mothers on the development of asthma targeted the mothers' personality characteristics, rather than emphasizing the possible psychological meanings of the asthma attack for the child. This research found that mothers of asthmatic children tend to be domineering, argumentative, controlling, overprotective, and passive–aggressive. Unfortunately, it was discovered that mothers of children with other chronic medical illnesses act the same way. So these characteristics may reflect the typical maternal response to chronic illness in a child, regardless of the type of illness. Mothers of sick children may end up being more controlling and protective. How do *you* act when someone you love is ill?

Finally, researchers observed that children with asthma tend to spend more time with their mothers than other children, so they concluded that a child's dependence on his or her mother causes asthma. Later, however, it was suggested that because children cannot predict when an asthma attack will occur, it makes sense for them to remain near someone who can help if their breathing worsens, namely, Mother. So another theory about how mothers cause asthma was debunked.

In reality, identifying the causes of a chronic illness is always a tricky business. Keep in mind that some connection or correlation between asthma and another factor does not itself prove that the other factor is a cause. Your mother could be genetically responsible for your asthma because it tends to run in families, but that's all we can say with certainty about your mother's having caused your asthma. And, of course, pointing a finger at your mother is just blaming your mother for your illness rather than blaming yourself.

Myth #5: "Don't worry, all children grow out of asthma."

Here's one you'll probably hear if your child has asthma. This myth serves to reassure anxious parents, but an unintended effect is to minimize the seriousness of the child's condition. Making this statement is like putting asthma in the same category as teething: children go through certain stages, and parents must endure the behavior until the stage ends. On the contrary, asthma symptoms are treated and controlled, not endured. All kinds of adverse effects are likely if a child's asthma remains untreated because the parent hopes the child will outgrow it. These effects may include impaired peer relationships, poor self-esteem, or increased dependence on others. Of course, another result of untreated asthma could be the death of the child.

It is true that around two-thirds of children with asthma will notice either a lessening or a remission of symptoms in puberty. No one really knows precisely why this happens. One idea is that the air passageways get larger as the child grows. Breathing is easier, because there is more room for air to flow into and out of the lungs. However, these changes do not mean that the child has outgrown asthma. Rather, the underlying respiratory disease is present, yet for some reason the symptoms have diminished. Unfortunately, these symptoms frequently return sometime during adulthood. In fact, we have seen some patients whose asthma returned after several decades of remission. So what happened? Did these people "catch" asthma again? Not really. For some reason the respiratory disease, present during all those years, was reactivated. Asthma can appear or reappear at any time of life, bringing along with it new life-functioning problems. That's one very good reason for the biopsychosocial approach to asthma: it helps you spot and react quickly to the more subtle social and psychological challenges that accompany physical symptoms.

Although it seems impossible to determine who will redevelop asthma as an adult after years of symptom-free living, there are some data to indicate which child's asthma will remit and which will not. One basic rule is that the earlier the asthma develops and the more severe the symptoms, the less likely the child will experience a remission. So, if uncontrollable asthma symptoms begin before the age of two years, you should not expect a reduction in symptoms. Furthermore, if the child continues to have symptoms into puberty, a remission is unlikely because symptom diminution occurs most often during puberty. While these rules can be reassuring, keep in mind that many children's asthma does not follow them.

Myth #6: "Move to Arizona. That'll cure your asthma."

Don't pack your bags for the desert of the Southwest without first taking steps to manage your symptoms well at home, no matter what your well-meaning friends may advise. Although some people do note a decrease in their symptoms after a move to a different climate, many of these people find their symptoms eventually return, because their lungs become responsive to new substances in the air. And some people find that their symptoms worsen after a move, and discover new allergies that they never had before.

Some families move because they want a new psychological climate, not a new meteorological climate.

> ১ One couple, Karen and Steven, decided to move to Utah from the Midwest. They acknowledged that the lower humidity and fewer molds would probably be better for Karen's asthma, but the real reason for the move was to get away from Steven's family, who worried constantly about Karen's health and sometimes seemed to treat her like an infant needing continuous care. Karen and Steven had grown tired of the persistent phone calls and visits, all beginning with the same question: "Are you okay?" Rather than continue to deal with this stress, they decided to put some distance between themselves and Steven's family. Although Karen discovered that the climate in Utah did not improve her asthma, she got more support from Steven because they stopped arguing about his family's treatment of her.

So, if you want to relocate to a new city, keep in mind that your in-laws may not follow you, but your asthma certainly will.

ASTHMA FUNDAMENTALS

This book is intended to help you cope better with your asthma and its effects on your life and on others around you. It is not intended to provide medical information. Several good books describe the symptoms, causes, and medical treatments for asthma, and you would be wise to read at least one of them to become fully informed (see the list in the Appendix at the end of this book for some recommendations). You may, in fact, wish to read several. New directions in asthma treatment are constantly being developed, and having an overview of the medical options available to you—from traditional Western medicine to ancient Eastern disciplines and modern herbalism and naturopathy—will help you and your health care providers make informed decisions that are right for you.

Even if you choose not to seek such information beyond your doctor's office, however, you should understand the fundamental physical aspects of the disease—what asthma is, the physical symptoms it may produce, and the potential triggers of an exacerbation. People who are mired in confusion about the physical illness of asthma can hardly be expected to address its attendant psychological and social problems. Ignorance about what's happening to your body can only keep you in constant fear—and that's not living well with asthma.

WHAT IS ASTHMA?

All asthma patients have one thing in common: their lungs are hypersensitive, or easily irritated, by specific circumstances. This lung overreaction causes the airways in the lungs, known as *bronchial tubes*, to narrow. This narrowing hinders movement of air both into and out of the lungs, making breathing difficult and labored. This narrowing is called an *asthma attack* or an *asthma exacerbation*. Remember that the narrowing of the airways is reversible. Sometimes the blockage or obstruction reverses by itself. More frequently, medications can successfully open the bronchial tubes.

INGREDIENTS OF AN ASTHMA ATTACK

Three things occur in the lungs to narrow the bronchial tubes. First, the muscles around the airways in the lungs tighten. Second, the membranes that line the airways become both inflamed and swollen. Finally, there is an increase in mucus secretion. Let's look at these ingredients one at a time.

Muscle Constriction

Everyone's bronchial tubes have muscles wrapped around them. By constricting and loosening, the muscles can change the size of the airway. When the muscles tighten, the airway opening gets smaller. As the muscles relax, the airway opening becomes larger. You cannot control these muscles; their movements work by reflex. Irritants such as cigarette smoke, gasoline fumes, perfume, and air pollution will cause everyone's muscles around the bronchial tube to constrict, narrowing the air passage. However, these muscles are hypersensitive in asthma patients and will constrict in response to a wider range of stimuli. As a result, the muscles may constrict not only to irritants but also to allergens, such as pollens, exercise, and cold air.

Inflammation

The inner membranes or walls that line the airways become inflamed and swollen during an asthma attack, further narrowing the size of the bronchial tube. The swelling is a result of the inflammation, because the membrane becomes filled with fluid and white blood cells. When you combine the muscle constriction on the outside of the bronchial tube with the inflammation and swelling of the inside membrane, the airways can become quite narrow.

Excess Mucus

A thin layer of mucus lines the bronchial tubes to lubricate air so that it will flow smoothly. However, mucus production increases dramatically during an asthma attack. Sometimes there is so much mucus that it creates a plug and clogs the airway. So the air you breathe not only must travel through narrowed bronchial tubes, but it also must pass through gobs of sticky mucus.

THE SYMPTOMS OF ASTHMA

Shortness of Breath

This symptom is the most common experienced by anyone with asthma. Many people describe it as "breathing through a straw." Other people feel as if their "chest is tight," as if there were tightly wrapped rubber bands around their chest. The circumstances under which people become short of breath vary depending on their asthma. Some people have trouble breathing during exercise, others experience it after inhaling smoke or pollen, while others need to ingest particular foods to become short of breath. Regardless of the triggering circumstances, all people with asthma seem to have trouble breathing.

The funny, and frustrating, thing about asthma is that you're not constantly short of breath. Most of the time your breathing may seem just fine. This waxing and waning is one of the defining elements of asthma: asthma is reversible, and so eventually the breathing troubles subside. However, this characteristic is also frustrating to people because it seems as if you can never predict when the shortness of breath is going to occur.

Wheezing

Not all people with asthma wheeze, but many do. The wheezing sound is caused by high-pitched vibrations as the stream of air passes through constricted airways. The wheezing sound can occur during both inhalation and exhalation and can be either loud or muted. This symptom makes asthma a noticeable illness. Most of the time asthma is invisible, and most people take their lungs and the work of breathing for granted. But wheezing is something other people can hear, so the asthma is readily noticed by them. For some persons with asthma, the wheezing sound is embarrassing because it serves to draw attention to them. For other people, wheezing provides a small amount of reassurance during an anxious time because it warns others that they're having trouble breathing and may need help.

Coughing

Like the wheezing sound, the symptom of coughing makes asthma visible to other people. Not all asthma patients cough, yet for some people cough is the primary symptom because they rarely wheeze. Patients whose primary symptom is coughing sometimes have difficulty with physicians, because they do not demonstrate the telltale wheeze of asthma. As a result, these physicians don't believe that the patient has asthma. While chronic cough can stem from a variety of sources, certainly asthma is one of them. In asthma, the cough can be the result of excessive mucus secretion or the spasms of the muscles surrounding the airways.

Mucus Production

Phlegm, spit, mucus, junk—call it what you will, most asthmatics have more than their share of this stuff. It can make sleeping, swallowing, talking, and simply breathing more difficult. Excess mucus is an unwelcome part of most asthma patients' lives.

Mucus production means that the person brings mucus up out of the airways and spits it out. You really aren't creating the mucus, but rather bringing it out of your lungs. Usually, mucus production is accompanied by a cough because coughing facilitates the movement of mucus up the air passageways. Although it can appear disgusting to others, most patients feel relieved and breathe better for a time after coughing up trapped mucus.

ASTHMA TRIGGERS

Figuring out what triggers an asthma attack for a specific person can be an exhausting task. While there is general agreement about the symptoms of asthma, it seems as if no two people are alike when it comes to triggers. Some people have allergies; others do not. Some people respond rapidly to cold air or exercise, while others have no trouble skiing. It is the wide range of potential asthma triggers that makes asthma such a complicated illness. Let's review some of the most common triggers of asthma.

Allergies

Not all asthmatics are allergic, and not everyone with allergies has asthma. Usually, no specific allergy trigger can be found in the majority of adults with asthma. If you and your doctor discover an allergy trigger for you, your asthma may be called *extrinsic asthma* because the trigger is external to you. The remainder of patients, without such well-defined external causes, suffer from *intrinsic asthma*. This distinction does not mean that intrinsic asthma is all in the patient's head. It just means that an external trigger cannot be found, and something internal likely precipitates asthma attacks.

People are not born with allergies. Allergies develop over a period of time in someone who is biologically disposed to developing them. For an allergy to develop, you need to be exposed repeatedly to a substance known as an *allergen*. The most common allergens include pollens, animal dander, dust, and molds. Repeated exposure to the allergen sensitizes a person's immune system. For those people with extrinsic asthma, the immune system becomes sensitive to one or more allergens, so that later contact causes the body to produce chemicals that irritate the already overreactive airways, prompting an asthma attack.

Scientists are now developing new medications aimed at stopping the effects of allergens. *Leukotriene inhibitors* are one of a variety of such drugs; they decrease the work of leukotrienes, which help trigger asthma attacks. Briefly, leukotrienes sense allergens and cause other molecules to be released to fight the allergen. Too many of these other molecules constrict your bronchial tubes. The idea behind these new medications is to decrease leukotriene activity so fewer molecules are released and your air passages remain open. You can take hope, therefore, that there are now medications designed to treat a cause of your asthma rather than just the symptoms.

Irritants

Irritants are also external triggers of asthma, but because they do not directly affect the immune system, they are not considered allergens. Irritants include cigarette smoke, gasoline fumes, perfume, cold air, and air pollution. They cause asthma symptoms by stimulating receptors in the nose and throat. These irritation receptors then excite the vagus nerve, which causes the muscles of the airways to constrict. As a result, the airways diminish in size, making it difficult to breathe. While everyone's vagus nerve is stimulated and airway muscles constrict when exposed to an irritant, you must remember as an asthmatic person, you have hyperreactive lungs, and the response of your airway muscles is even greater.

Infections

Many patients with asthma will say that their symptoms started after a cold. In fact, an upper respiratory infection produces many of the symptoms associated with asthma. The inner membranes of the bronchial tubes become inflamed, reducing the size of the airways. Mucus is also produced, sometimes blocking the airways. Having asthma, you are handicapped further because your lungs are already primed toward muscle constriction, inflammation, and mucus production. This predisposition can make the infection even worse. No one really knows why some patients develop asthma after an upper respiratory infection. For that matter, it is unclear why someone with asthma is more prone to these kinds of infections.

Exercise

For many people asthma symptoms are triggered by exercise. So what is the logical thing to do if physical exertion causes you to become short of breath and wheeze? Slow down and stop exercising. Unfortunately, although this response makes sense, taking it easy is not the best thing to do for your body. For example, you may gain weight, which makes breathing more difficult. You may become depressed and irritable, which can create family tension and then prompt an asthma attack. So what can you do? Well, you can exercise with asthma even if you have found it triggers symptoms. Depending on your physical conditioning and pretreating with medications prior to exercise, most activities can be enjoyed. However, strenuous, continuous exercise is frequently not recommended because the air you are breathing rapidly into and out of your mouth is dry and cold. This kind of air typically triggers an asthma attack. When you are breathing normally, air can be both warmed and humidified before it reaches the lung airways. Long periods of energetic exercise do not allow that process to occur. So, if you want to exercise with fewer worries, find a sport that involves brief episodes of activity followed by a rest period. Golf, softball, football, and tennis can all be enjoyed by persons with asthma. Swimming may be all right because the air you breathe is humidified and there is water all around, but chlorine may be problematic, so pools may not be your best choice. However, if you remain fixed on the goal of becoming a long-distance runner, good conditioning and consultation with your physician about medication pretreatment are necessary. (For more details on exercise, see Chapter 10.)

Psychological Factors

Asthma is not all in your head, but your thoughts, feelings, and relationships with others can affect your asthma. For example, many people find that stress at work or at home can make them short of breath. A child who does not listen to anything can eventually infuriate a parent. The ensuing anger causes the parent to constrict all of his or her muscles and to begin breathing rapidly. This muscle tension and rapid, shallow breathing can then precipitate an asthma attack. Other people find that strong feelings, such as anxiety, prompt symptoms of asthma. Many people with asthma become nervous and panicky during an asthma attack; it's frightening to feel as if you're suffocating. In turn, these anxious feelings seem to worsen asthma symptoms. Finally, some asthma patients discover that one or more relationships worsen their asthma. The other person can be overly solicitous, critical, or demanding, attitudes that make the asthmatic person increasingly tense or angry, thereby triggering an asthma attack. As with all asthma triggers, the specific thoughts, feelings, or relationships that precipitate an asthma attack vary from person to person. You need to identify which psychological factors seem to apply to you.

How well you live with asthma depends in great part on your willingness and ability to take into account the complicated biological, psychological, and social factors involved in managing the physical disease. If that sounds like a formidable task, what it really boils down to is getting to know yourself better. Becoming fully aware of how asthma is affecting you in body, mind, and spirit makes you an ideal collaborator for your physician and gives you the power to adapt to life with asthma rather than merely accept the restrictions of a chronic disease.

No doubt, one of the first changes you've noticed is in how you view yourself now that your body is behaving differently. Changes in body image resulting from a diagnosis of asthma can make you feel isolated, alienated from yourself as well as from others. Understanding what you're going through—and that the millions of others with asthma are going through it right along with you—can spare you much psychological and social pain. The next four chapters describe how many people respond to a diagnosis of asthma—starting with changes in body image—and offer some flexible tools for learning to live better with this illness. As you'll see, living better with asthma means a lot more than just breathing easier.

৯ PART II

. . . BUT YOU MAY FEEL ALONE

‿ Chapter 2

"My Body Feels Out of Control!"

The most compelling evidence we have that asthma is more than a physical disease is how it changes the way you feel about your body. Your immediate reaction to the diagnosis of asthma may have been shock, surprise, or even relief. But no matter how long ago you received the news, you probably remember that your relationship with your body quickly changed. Suddenly, breathing, that most unconscious of actions, was pushed to the forefront of your consciousness. Actions that you never thought twice about performing had to be reconsidered. No longer could you take your body for granted; it was now an important focus of your life. These changes in your physical functioning can elicit strong feelings about your body, significant changes in your body image. Joan, a forty-year-old mother of two, explains:

> ‿ "I used to exercise every now and then, but not very often. I tried to prepare foods that are good for me and my family—not too much fried chicken, which I love—and I got plenty of sleep. You know, I tried to take good care of myself. But after being sick with the flu, I was short of breath all the time. I didn't know what was happening to me. Then my doctor diagnosed me with asthma. I was devastated. I felt like my body was betraying me. I wanted to

play with the kids, but after only a few minutes I was out of breath. I had to sit down, and they'd be tugging at me, pleading for me to play more with them. I felt like a terrible mother. I just couldn't play with the kids, and I was angry.

"Weeks later I realized that I couldn't stay angry and upset with my body all my life. I mean, what other body do I have? So, I talked with my doctor about what I could do, and she suggested an exercise program. After thinking about different exercises, I started swimming every other day; I'm not sensitive to chlorine, and it's something I could do in the winter. I found myself feeling better, about both my asthma and my body. Also, my stamina increased, and it's easier now for me to play with the kids. It's not like before the asthma, but it's certainly better. While I still get angry with my body when I don't feel well, at least it seems that my body is usually cooperating with me to remain healthy."

As Joan's story illustrates, changes in body image caused by asthma can have sweeping effects—on your feelings, your behavior, and, in turn, your physical control over your asthma. But there is plenty you can do to offset any negative impact. In this chapter we'll examine how and why asthma changes your body image and what you can do about it. A changing body image is not only one of the first nonphysical issues that asthma will hand you but also one of the most enduring. Therefore, it's important to begin addressing it now.

YOU VERSUS YOUR BODY

After her diagnosis of asthma, Joan felt betrayed and angry because it seemed as if she had lost control over her body and her ability to do things that really matter to her, such as playing with her children. She began to experience her body as separate from herself, as if it had a mind of its own and its own motivations. Joan did not want asthma, but her body had forced it on her. She did not want to be prevented from doing things she enjoyed, but her body frequently reminded her about the limitations asthma placed on her life.

Sometimes you may feel that your body is your enemy, as if you're engaged in a struggle of wills between your wishes and those of your body. For many people this struggle becomes increasingly competitive and filled with strong emotions. "It seems like I'm at war with my body," Fred observed. "I want to force it to do things that it doesn't want to do. We have battles every day. Sometimes I win, sometimes I lose. I'm the big loser when my body sends me to the hospital. But that's becoming less frequent because I'm working closely with my doctor to better control my asthma." The most difficult aspect of such a war is, to paraphrase Pogo, we have met the enemy, and he is us. You cannot run away from your body. It is, as Fred stated, important to work as a partner with your doctor, but first you need to be sure your mind and body are partners.

Calling a Truce

How can you call a truce and accept your body as an equal partner? Sustaining a fruitful relationship is a lifelong task, but there are steps you can take to start the peace talks. The following suggestions are some body-wise rules to live by; they will be developed more fully later in this chapter and throughout the book.

1. ***Recognize that you have only one body.*** This idea may seem obvious on the face of it, but, as Joan said, sometimes we need to remind ourselves of this irrefutable fact. There's no way to replace the body you have, so you might as well start working with it rather than against it.

2. ***Try not to deny that you have asthma.*** Accepting your body also means accepting your asthma, because that is where your asthma resides. Deny that you have asthma and the struggles with your body will continue. By always pushing yourself, without thinking about your breathing, you force your body to remind you that you have asthma through symptoms such as dyspnea (shortness of breath) or bronchial spasms. Some people need several visits to the hospital emergency room before they begin listening to their body.

3. *Get up and actively negotiate with your body.* Don't just throw in the towel because you believe your body rebels against activity. Many people resign themselves to living a sedentary life, sitting in recliners and watching television. Acceptance of your asthma should not mean resignation and defeat. Living with your asthma does not mean inactivity. Rather, it means creating those circumstances that allow you to live an energetic life. Pace yourself when you're not feeling particularly well. Understand what things trigger your asthma and try to avoid or minimize exposure to them. Consistently do peak flow metering so you can anticipate whether you may be ripe for an asthma attack, and then take the steps to keep it from happening. If you can listen to your body, you can negotiate with it.

4. *Become a partner with your doctor in managing your asthma.* Be detectives, and the two of you can discover factors that worsen your asthma. Learn about the effects of different medications on your body. Become an informed patient and make important decisions about your asthma with your doctor rather than just complying with recommendations. By understanding your illness, you can regain some control over your body, and that sense of control can help you call a truce with your body.

5. *Use exercise to reintegrate your body with yourself.* During any form of exercise, you and your body are working together in harmony toward a goal. No longer do you feel at war. This sense of cooperation is supported further by knowing that a body in good shape allows you to be more physically active. Chapter 10 gives specifics on exercising when you have asthma.

6. *Learn to deflect comments such as, "That's funny, you don't look sick."* Your body may be where the asthma resides, but the asthma itself remains concealed. Asthma is usually an invisible illness (though there are exceptions, described later in this chapter), so when others are told you have asthma they may respond with insensitive dismissal. You know how asthma has changed your body and your body image, so don't let such remarks convince you that it's nothing. Take such dismissals as an opportunity to help people understand that many chronic illnesses, including asthma, are not obvious to the naked eye. Explain that you might not look sick at that particular time, but there are moments during which you gasp for air. You'll be surprised to find that such explanations not only educate others about asthma but also help make asthma real and manageable for you.

Keep these commandments in mind, and your body image will get a healthy boost. It's a complicated image, though, made up of all the thoughts, impressions, and feelings you have about your physical being. Everyone has a body, healthy or ill, a body image, shaped by a complex mix of influences over many years. Understanding how body image develops over a lifetime can help you maintain a positive body image despite the changes wrought by asthma.

DEVELOPMENT OF BODY IMAGE

Jay has had asthma consistently for twenty-five years but emits an air of confident vitality as he goes about the business of an active life. Allie was diagnosed a year ago; when she looks in the mirror, she can't believe she's seeing the same person who is in the picture on her dresser taken at about the same time. Sid, whose moderate asthma has come and gone several times since he was five, walks with the stooped gait of someone much older. Asthma can have a wide range of effects on your body image, depending on when the disease begins, how it is managed and treated, and how others treat you. Can you recognize your own body image influences in the following pages?

Infancy

An infant's primary means of contact is through the body. The warmth of the mother's breast, the secure grip of the father's arms, the gentle rocking in a chair by a grandmother all convey important messages to the baby. The infant develops a sense of trust in the environment as well as a beginning impression of what his or her body is. When an infant is diagnosed with asthma, the parents can be worried, sad, or resentful. These feelings are felt by the infant through the parents' bodies. Muscular tension conveys the parents' concern to the infant. These feelings permeate the baby's environment, and every medical procedure can heighten parents' anxiety, which is then conveyed to the baby. The infant is thus left feeling insecure about both the environment and his or her body.

Childhood

Months later the baby begins to sit, stand, and crawl. These advances help the infant learn more about the position of different body parts as well as their size. Toward the beginning of the third year, the child knows how he or she looks to others based on repeated reactions by them. For example, a girl may know that others respond positively to her long, full hair. A boy may know that he is bigger and stronger than other children his age because of the responses of others. By this process children learn what aspects of their bodies other people respond to positively or negatively, and these data are integrated into their body image.

As in infancy, however, asthma can have a negative impact. A child with asthma may learn, for example, that physical activity provokes a parent to ask the child to stop playing so hard and do something more sedentary. The child discovers that physical exertion is to be avoided because there is something wrong with his or her body.

Linda, the mother of four-year-old Sarah, who has asthma, describes well how parents influence their children's body image:

&ern; "When Sarah was diagnosed with asthma last year, my husband and I were terrified. Now, I know we're overprotective of Sarah, but I still don't like it when she's on the playground. I tell her to slow down, not run so fast, or stop playing rough with the other kids. I'm just so worried that she's going to have an asthma attack that I don't want her to play so hard. She complains about it, but her health is so important to me."

Sarah confirms her mother's impressions when talking about things she likes to do: "I like drawing, painting, and playing with dolls. I'm a very good painter and do lots of them for Mommy, Daddy, Grandma, Grandpa. I don't like the playground that much. The boys always climb and swing so fast, and I can't climb too much, because then I can't breathe. But I'm the best painter in my whole class!"

Parents' concern and involvement are important, yet sometimes the message they convey to their children is that their body is something that limits their wishes and goals; their body is different from those of other children, and they must play differently. With time the child may begin to resent both the limit-setting parents and his or her own negative body image.

When a child enters school, a new set of people and values becomes important. Teachers, other adults, and, most important, other children begin to react to the child, and these reactions affect body image. There is a pressing need to fit in, and if the child appears different for any reason, the effects on body image and sense of self can be profound. Ryan, age ten, explains the importance of peer relations on body image:

> "I do pretty well in school, mostly A's and B's. Science is my favorite subject 'cause I like learning about dinosaurs. The only time I have a little trouble is at recess. I don't like running around too much, because I don't want to get out of breath. Sometimes the other boys make fun of me, but I'm scared of my chest getting real hard and tight. I'll go on the swings and the jungle gym, but playing ball's real hard. I'm not a sissy like the other boys think. I'm just scared of my chest and breathing."

Adolescence

When the child becomes an adolescent, body image must change dramatically. The development of secondary sexual characteristics, such as breasts or facial hair, needs to be integrated into the previously developed body image. Now the body image becomes infused with sexuality, and, once again, the reactions of others are an important determinant of body image. For example, a girl who develops breasts earlier than others in her peer group may find herself teased by boys. This ridicule can prompt the girl to feel embarrassed by her breasts, viewing them as undesirable parts of herself. She may then try to hide them by wearing loose-fitting clothes or, more seriously, undergo cosmetic surgery as an adult. Asthma creates particular difficulties for adolescents because it can exacerbate concerns about sexuality. The physical exertion that adolescents typically associate with sex is viewed as a new challenge, another scary bodily activity that can prompt an asthma attack. Such concerns can cause some teenagers to avoid close relationships with opposite-sex peers, fearing that such relations inevitably will result in some kind of sexual behavior, activity that must be avoided at all costs. Julie, age sixteen, describes these fears:

> "All the boys I know want sex. It's really what's on their mind. And I'm just not interested in that. Love belongs in a marriage, and that's where I want to find it. So I don't have much to do with most boys. I try to dress down, you know. Baggy, loose shirt and pants. I don't like to attract too much attention. Also, with my asthma I'm worried that I might have an asthma attack. I mean, there's a lot of moving going on when you make love. And I don't want to end up in a hospital. I don't mind having mainly girlfriends right now. But a boyfriend, no way!"

Although same-sex friendships are important during adolescence, Julie notes that her anxious body image affects her relationships with boys, another important aspect of adolescence, despite her attempts to minimize it.

Early Adulthood

Most people believe that their body image reaches the most positive point when they're in the early adulthood years. During that time they think their body is its most attractive and functioning best. Sometimes the wish to maintain this splendid body image is so strong that the presence of asthma simply cannot be admitted, seen typically as a defect to be avoided. Cindy, at age twenty-one, avoids her asthma with mixed results:

&> "I enjoy being outdoors. I work hard in an office, and whenever I have a chance I'm outdoors. So I ski every weekend during the winter, and I bike when the weather's nice. But I don't do that stuff just for fun. I'm real competitive and ski hard and bike hard. Otherwise, it's not enjoyable. Sure I have asthma, but I'm not going to let that stop me from playing. And, yes, sometimes I have difficulty breathing when I'm doing these things. I've even had to go to the emergency room, I don't know, five or six times. But I'm not going to stop competing, and I'm not going to do something like pretreating before I go out. I'm young and active. You can forget about that asthma stuff."

Cindy's denial of her asthma admittedly has had negative consequences at times, yet she persists in rejecting this aspect of her body. That's how powerful the need to maintain an impressive body image can be.

How would you describe *your* adult body image? If you've had asthma since childhood, how did the disease shape your body image then?

Middle and Old Age

Body image continues to change as people get older. Middle age brings with it a conflict between the wish to deny the aging process and the realities of a changing appearance and declining physical stamina. It's hard to accept the loss of a youthful body, especially when our society values it so highly. Some people never accept this loss and pursue rigorous exercise regimens and sometimes plastic surgery to stem the inevitable bodily changes. Physical activity is certainly important to everyone and should continue at any age. But attempts to regain past beauty are obviously doomed to failure. Fortunately, most people resolve this conflict by remaking their body image so it's more consistent with the reality of a middle-aged body.

For a person with asthma, however, previous struggles with body image can make this conflict protracted. Even if you settled any problems with endurance and physical exertion years ago, any age-related decline in stamina is bound to create opportunities for new resentment and bitterness. Mike, age fifty-three, describes these feelings:

> &❦ "I've had asthma all my life, and it's been very difficult to control. Even pretreating before exercise provided only some relief. So I found myself avoiding many things that required consistent physical exertion. I never got into the running craze or anything like that. I play a lot of tennis but rarely go for the ball on difficult returns. Why waste the energy? So I don't think I ever played up to my potential. I wasn't too happy about it, but that's life. Now I find myself losing a step or two more when I play, and I'm really angry about it. I know it's because I'm getting older—everyone else is too—but, heck, I've never played the way I knew I could, and now I'm playing even worse. Why couldn't I have just tried to return the hard shots? Because I have asthma and my body is different and difficult. Maybe I should just give up the whole thing and take up golf!"

Shortly, we'll explore the mechanisms by which body image exerts such enduring effects. But first, it's important to acknowledge the psychological effects of one bodily change that you may encounter in the course of asthma treatment.

WHEN THE INVISIBLE BECOMES VISIBLE: BODY IMAGE AND ORAL STEROIDS

Usually no one can simply look at you and see that you have a chronic respiratory problem needing consistent monitoring and treatment. There is, however, one circumstance that frequently creates dramatic changes in body appearance. When asthma is so difficult to control that long-term oral steroid use is required, a wide range of side effects may occur (these changes do not develop with short-term bursts of oral steroids or with inhaled steroids). Particularly distressing to many people are the substantial weight gain and fat redistribution accompanying long-term use of oral steroids. Betty, a thirty-one-year-old, single woman, talks about her forty-pound weight gain:

   • "I just eat, eat, eat. I'm always hungry, and I'm never satisfied. And now look at me: I never had this flab on my back and arms. My face has also changed; it's round like a basketball. I look in the mirror and don't recognize myself. It's terrible. I don't go on dates anymore, because no one would want me."

The change in Betty's face that so distresses her is one of the earliest side effects of long-term steroid use and is described by doctors as a "moon face." Oral steroids also stimulate the appetite and, as Betty attests, a significant weight gain usually ensues. Finally, fat is redistributed, becoming localized in the back, while the legs become thin and seem withered. All these changes in body appearance make most people feel very distressed, anxious, and sometimes depressed. Karen describes this dismay:

   • "My asthma has been difficult to control, so my doctor suggested steroid tablets. Since then I've gained sixty pounds, and it's all in my face, chest, and back. I don't recognize myself when I look in the mirror. Whose face is that? I ask myself. That's not me. This is not me. I don't understand it. I can't stand looking in the mirror or looking at myself. I can't go out with other people anymore. I'm a blimp! I wouldn't want to be seen with someone who looks like me. Why would anyone else? So I stay at home most of the time. At first, people used to call, wanting to go out to eat or to the movies. But I'd always say no. Now most of them don't even bother to call."

Many of the physical changes undergone by Betty and Karen diminish when oral steroids are reduced or discontinued, but steroid tapers take a long time to accomplish and risk flare-ups of asthma symptoms. For this reason, it would be wiser for both women to accept their bodies as they are now. But Karen clings so desperately to her past body image that she does not even recognize herself in a mirror. The price she has paid is a self-imposed exile.

HOW BODY IMAGE WORKS ON THE MIND

Obviously, body image influences a person's behavior. Sarah and Ryan prefer not to play too hard at the playground. Julie avoids boys, partly because she fears the physical exertion accompanying any kind of sexual behavior. Cindy refrains from thinking about her asthma and continues to compete in sports despite the occasional emergency room visit. And Betty and Karen remain isolated at home, preferring that others not see their changes in appearance. Their body image is dictating some of their behavior because it is having a profound impact on how these people feel about themselves. Body image can give rise to many unwelcome feelings, including poor self-confidence and self-esteem, anxiety, depression, shame, and resentment.

There is a close connection between how we view ourselves and how we view our bodies. In part, this relationship stems from the fact that our most rudimentary sense of self is as a body, independent from the outside world. You can see this process when infants begin to delight in the discovery that the hand in front of them is their own, which they can control and move. So, our body is closely tied to our self-experience, and any problems or deficiencies in body image can create strong negative feelings. Karen, for one, is so mortified by her body's appearance that she tries urgently to keep the image in the mirror from affecting her, saying repeatedly, "That person is not me," but such efforts do not diminish her feelings of humiliation. Similarly, Mike resents that his asthma precluded him from ever playing tennis to his potential. He feels betrayed by a body that made him act old before his time, and now that he is older, the simmering anger and resentment are beginning to boil over.

How you perceive your body to be functioning also influences your self-confidence and self-esteem. When your body is working well, you frequently take it for granted. You don't need to consider it when making decisions about whether to go to the supermarket, to visit with friends, or to play with your children. However, after you are diagnosed with asthma, body functioning begins to play a prominent role in even the simplest of decisions. Are you breathing well enough to visit a supermarket and push a cart laden with groceries? Is it all right to ask your friends not to wear perfume because the scent might trigger an asthma attack? Do you risk becoming short of breath by playing vigorously with the kids? Will other people think that you're hideous because of your weight? These questions affect not only your activities but your self-confidence: Are you able to do the things you want? Must you always be cautious and wary of your body, other people, and the environment? After a while that vigilance becomes a heavy burden. Then, your self-confidence and self-esteem drop, particularly if you find yourself more and more limited by your ever-present fears and anxieties. In turn, your behavior alters, and the cycle continues.

LIVING BETTER WITH YOUR BODY IMAGE

Joan said at the beginning of this chapter that she could not stay upset and angry with her body for the rest of her life, because it was the only body she had. She's right. You can allow your negative body image to adversely affect your life, limit your activities, and drain your self-confidence, or you can begin to develop a new body image that includes the asthma yet provides you with the freedom to enjoy life. Here's how.

Exercise

Many people with asthma believe that they should not exercise or pursue any strenuous activity. Nothing could be further from the truth. Exercise is helpful in so many ways that it is a cornerstone of biopsychosocial treatment. It resolves the conflicts between your body and your mind, it increases your physical fitness, and it boosts your self-esteem. All these benefits for only thirty minutes a day!

Although asthma is sometimes triggered by exercise, this problem can be overcome by pretreating with medications before you begin your exercise. You can then begin any number of physical activities that will allow you to improve your body image and your outlook. Some activities such as yoga and meditation attempt directly to reconcile conflicts between body and mind. Other physical activities, such as sports, exercise, or dance classes, allow you to experience your body positively rather than always focusing on its deficiencies. Starting new physical activities also increases your self-confidence, because you will be successful at doing something new despite your asthma. Some people even begin a competitive sport, such as golf or tennis, and their self-worth rises with each success in their new and challenging endeavor. So talk to your doctor about physical activities that might be best for you. Start something new and interesting; you will quickly begin feeling better about your body and yourself.

What Your Significant Other Can Do

Betty and Karen may have gone off on the wrong track when they anticipated (and exaggerated) others' reactions to their changes in appearance, but beneath their behavior is an incontrovertible fact: your body image is shaped not only by how you perceive your body and its functioning but also by the responses of others. When you think that people are staring at you because of your moon face, it reinforces your negative image of your face and discourages you from going outside again. Obviously, then, your spouse or lover can play a very important role in your living better with your body.

Your spouse can help you remember that body changes are an inevitable result of asthma. There will be times when you want to forget that you have asthma and again hold on to your body as it used to be, but your spouse can comfort and reassure you that you're still the same person despite the physical changes. Do things that you both enjoy doing. Find new activities that you both can learn together. Isn't there something that you've always wanted to do but haven't gotten around to? You can view any asthma exacerbation not only as a call for medical treatment but also as an opportunity to decide that now is the right time to try new things.

Living with your new body image is easier when your spouse can help you realize that not only are you the same person but also your marriage can endure asthma. Jeffrey describes how he helped both himself and his wife overcome their anxieties about her body:

> ह "When Sally was diagnosed with asthma, I wasn't sure what to do. I mean, I wasn't sure what she could or couldn't do. I was scared and worried; I didn't want to cause an asthma attack. But we had a good sex life before she was diagnosed with asthma, and it was important to both of us. I didn't want that to end because of her asthma. So we read about sex and asthma [see Chapter 7] and spent a lot of time just touching, hugging, and caressing before making love. We discovered that asthma didn't mean we couldn't make love; we just changed it a little from before. It was still enjoyable for both of us, and now Sally and I aren't nearly so worried or concerned. I still love Sally and find her desirable and attractive. I also think it's helped Sally feel good about her body and herself, that asthma was not going to keep us physically apart."

For most couples sex conveys love, affection, and respect for each other. It also communicates acceptance of and desire for one another's bodies. If you are angry, unhappy, or resentful about your body and have a poor body image, your spouse's behavior can quickly change your perception, particularly within the private, intimate, and trusted context of lovemaking.

Avoiding Triggers without Retreating from the World

As mentioned earlier, it's always helpful to work with your doctor so you can better understand the triggers of your asthma, such as allergies, infections, environmental irritants, and weather changes. By minimizing exposure to these triggers you can regain some control over your body. If household cleaners prompt your asthma symptoms, avoid such substances by negotiating to have your spouse do the housecleaning while you take on another chore. Asthma frequently forces spouses to shift household responsibilities, and these negotiations can focus on helping you avoid symptom triggers. If cigarette smoke and perfume produce your asthma symptoms, begin to talk to your family and friends about your need for a fume-free environment. By continuing to socialize with others, you will feel that your body is not a giant obstacle that interferes with all your relationships.

If you're among the many people who find it difficult to ask for a fume-free environment because you're embarrassed by drawing attention to your asthma and also feel you're infringing on the rights of others, remember that you also have a right to socialize in an environment that will not trigger your asthma. Also keep in mind that you will be talking to family and friends, not total strangers, who most likely will be receptive to your need to eliminate cigarette smoke, perfume, or other irritants.

If you still find it hard to ask for such changes, practicing what you will say can be a great help. Rehearse to yourself how to approach others in a way that seems comfortable and natural to you: Keep it short and simple? Inject a little humor? Make a call ahead of time, or wait until the situation is at hand? Anticipate the responses you're likely to get so you'll be prepared for your own reaction to them. They're bound to be much less critical than you anticipate. To gain assurance of being heard, try this time-honored method: put your request in terms of your own needs while acknowledging how the other person may feel ("I know this may be an imposition, but I feel . . . " rather than inadvertently blaming with a "you" statement).

If such practice still does not stem your anxiety, assertiveness training may be helpful. Rest assured that this problem is so pervasive that libraries and bookstores are full of whole books on the subject. Assertiveness training can help you not only improve your body image but also fulfill other needs imposed by asthma.

Making Little Changes in Your Appearance

A final practical technique for resolving problems with body image is to make little changes to your physical appearance, particularly if you have gained weight because of long-term oral steroid use. This may sound like obvious advice, but when self-esteem is low due to a damaged body image, it's difficult to remember the disproportionately positive effect on your psyche of making a simple superficial change. Try a new clothing style. Experiment with a new hairstyle or new makeup that minimizes the weight gain in your face. Try a beard or mustache on for size.

Remember that no one's body is perfect. We can all point to something about our bodies that we don't like. Sure, making changes is hard when you feel you look terrible. But you must live with your body, so actively do things that will improve your appearance. Who knows? Maybe you'll keep the beard or hairstyle after you've stopped the steroids and lost the weight.

Changing Thoughts about Your Body

If you try these suggestions and still feel bad about your body, a more focused approach may be necessary. One useful strategy to help you develop a positive physical image and reconcile with your body involves changing the thoughts associated with your body. With the help of a psychologist, Karen changed her thoughts about her body and reconciled with both her body and her friends. This cognitive process could be used by the other people described in this chapter who were having problems with body image; in fact, it can be used to modify many perceptions and beliefs that are hindering your chances of living well with asthma, as we'll describe in the following two chapters. Here is how Karen used the technique:

1. The first step in this process requires monitoring the thoughts associated with your body. Karen listed the following thoughts: "I look grotesque, and everyone will be repulsed by my appearance. I'm too embarrassed to go out, and everyone will point at me and laugh at me. I can't go to the supermarket because I'll just die if anyone sees me."

2. The second step requires evaluating the assumptions and implications of these thoughts. Many of these thoughts include a cognitive error. For example, Karen's belief that she is grotesque and everyone will be repulsed by her is an exaggeration. Her idea that everyone who sees her will laugh at her is emo-

tional reasoning. Finally, her belief that she will die if anyone recognizes her at the supermarket is both jumping to an inappropriate conclusion and exaggerating.

3. The final step toward developing a better body image involves presenting rational counterarguments to such cognitive errors and stating more helpful interpretations. As Karen illustrates:

> ॐ "I may be overweight, but I'm not grotesque or repugnant. I mean, people won't get sick when they see me. I'm just overweight because my asthma is difficult to control. And people certainly aren't going to stop what they're doing to point at me and laugh. Most really won't care how I look; they have more important things to do. So, now, I'm visiting again with friends and slowly going out to restaurants and movies. And it's been all right. Sometimes people do stare at me, but it doesn't last very long, and it really doesn't bother me that much. I mean, I'm with my friends who really like me, regardless of how I look. I guess I just needed to learn to be comfortable with my body before I could like myself. And allow other people to like me too."

It's important to note that Karen says she needed to accept herself before allowing other people to like her too. It was Karen who refused to go out with her friends. They continued to accept her and stopped calling only when she persistently declined their invitations. Should you ever decide to isolate yourself out of fear that your friends can't accept the way you now look, reread what one of Karen's friends, Shirley, had to say:

> ॐ "Sure, Karen gained weight, but she was still Karen. I wanted to see her because she's a funny, caring person whom I liked being with. I noticed her weight gain, but she wasn't this grotesque person. I wasn't embarrassed to be with her. And when she called to get together, I was pleased as punch. It's hard to make good friends, and I didn't want to lose her."

Sometimes, but not always, we build the biggest obstacles to living well with asthma by ourselves. Certainly, Karen's refusal to see others stemmed from her own misconceptions, not really the reactions of her friends. It took some time for Karen to overcome these ideas and allow others to both support and enjoy her. Karen says it well: if you can accept your body, you can accept yourself. And once you accept both your body and yourself, you can give others the chance to express their understanding, compassion, and concern. Their support will help you live better with your asthma and your body.

ঌ Chapter 3

"Of Course I'm Upset; My Life Is Ruined!"

Feelings are a part of everyday life. In fact, you can think of them as the spice that makes life vibrant and compelling. Sorrow, happiness, fright, and glee provide texture and energy to each day. Some people even seek events that will heighten a specific emotion, a major reason for the success of both horror movies and drug abuse. Living with asthma every day seriously influences your feelings. For many people, asthma seems to generate too much spice, intense sadness, crippling anxiety, or severe despair. Life becomes unpleasant, leaving a terrible taste in their mouths. Eddie, a forty-nine-year-old husband and father of four, describes this unpleasant taste and how he made life less spicy and more agreeable to him:

> ঌ "It's always been hard raising four children. My wife and I are constantly on the go. If we're not playing referee when the kids are fighting, we're driving them to soccer practice, guitar lessons, or some other place. There's always something to do or someplace to go. It's hard work. But my wife and I had an agreement. Every Saturday night, we got a baby-sitter and went country dancing. We used to go dancing all the time before we got married, and when the kids got old enough for a babysitter, we decided we needed time away from them and started dancing again on Satur-

days. It was great fun until I got asthma. Then, I couldn't dance like I used to. The smoke made it even more difficult to breathe. And just dancing became hard work too.

"I became really depressed, saying to myself that I was a terrible husband because I couldn't do something my wife really enjoyed, thinking that she would leave me since I couldn't dance anymore. I mean, she's real attractive, and other men at the bar, good dancers too, would want to dance with her. Why would she want to be with me when she could be with one of them? I know now that it didn't make sense, but back then it sure seemed to.

"Well, I've got a real smart wife, and she noticed that I was down in the dumps. After a while she just kept asking me what was wrong. I would say nothing at first, but she stayed on top of me. Finally I told her that the country dancing wasn't any fun anymore, what with the fast pace and the smoke. I also told her that I felt like a terrible husband, that she would prefer being with someone else. Well, she straightened me out right away and told me I was totally wrong in my thinking—that she was interested in spending time with me, away from the kids, not just in the dancing. I guess I was depressed and down on myself. I forgot the real reason we went dancing. Now, we go to all kinds of places on Saturday night—dinner, movies, baseball games. In fact, I'm starting to exercise more regularly so we can go dancing again; maybe we can find a smoke-free dance hall! And our marriage is better than ever."

Eddie's wife taught him that feelings are controllable and that the power to control his emotions was his. How did she teach him this very important lesson? By correcting his *perception* of events. Events do not cause sadness, anxiety, or anger. Rather, how we interpret these events—the thoughts that accompany events in our lives—determines whether we are severely affected by them. It wasn't Eddie's dancing problems that caused his sadness and anxiety but his interpretation of these problems. When Eddie's asthma suddenly made it difficult for him to enjoy dancing, causing him to think that he wasn't a good husband, that he wasn't tending to his wife's needs, and that she would leave him for someone else, Eddie felt depressed and worthless. Luckily, his wife took notice, forced him to say what was on his mind, and then corrected his faulty beliefs. That helped him feel less depressed and more relaxed with his wife, and opened him up to developing new ways to enjoy Saturday night.

As we discussed in Chapter 2, asthma can immediately make you feel as if your body is no longer in your control. As time goes on and your mind registers the many changes the disease brings, you may begin to feel as if your entire life is no longer in your control. Little wonder that you end up feeling depressed or anxious, sad or angry. Fortunately, as Eddie discovered, you can to some extent control your emotional reactions to your new life with asthma. Sometimes it's your head that is getting you into trouble, and it's your head that can get you out of it. In this chapter we'll introduce you to some self-checks for short-circuiting overly negative feelings. And because a certain amount of emotional stress is inevitable, we'll offer a few preventive measures that you can make an ongoing part of your life.

THE THINKING–FEELING CONNECTION

Eddie illustrates the chain by which the thoughts that accompany events cause feelings: I cannot go country dancing because of my asthma (initial event); I'm a terrible husband, so my wife will find another man more interesting and attractive (thoughts and beliefs); I'm worthless and helpless (emotion). Eddie's conversations with his wife corrected his faulty beliefs, drastically changing his emotional reaction without altering the initial event: I cannot go country dancing because of my asthma (initial event); although I cannot go dancing, there are other pleasant and desirable things we can do together as a couple (thoughts and beliefs); I'm happy and content (emotion).

Certainly, we are able to avoid some events that we know might bring unhappiness, anxiety, or anger. For example, adhering to a medication regimen will preclude an asthma attack, which would have created much anxiety. It would be unrealistic, however, to expect to prevent all unpleasant things from happening to us. We are much more capable of altering our thoughts and beliefs about events, so we might as well concentrate on that. It is, after all, the only sure way to control unpleasant feelings.

There are no happy or sad events. How we look at and think about these events will determine whether they are happy or sad.

Although we all have our own way of viewing events based on background and experience, there also appear to be common faulty beliefs associated with specific feelings. Which of the following do you believe?

⋗ BELIEFS THAT MAKE YOU SAD AND DEPRESSED

1. I am never going to be happy, because I have asthma.
2. I am inferior and flawed because of my asthma.
3. I am an awful person because my asthma won't let me clean the house [or fulfill any other responsibility or participate in any other activity].
4. I'm going to die soon because I have asthma.
5. My wife [or anyone important] won't love me because of my asthma.

⋗ BELIEFS THAT MAKE YOU NERVOUS AND WORRIED

1. I can't survive with asthma.
2. My husband [or anyone important] must be around me all the time in case I have an asthma attack.
3. I need to be sure that I won't have an asthma attack before I go bicycling [or do any other activity].
4. I cannot leave my hometown, because only my doctor can help me.

⋗ BELIEFS THAT MAKE YOU ANGRY

1. I will never have an asthma attack.
2. I can do anything; asthma's not going to stop me.
3. My asthma must be caused by my parents.
4. Why did I have to get asthma?
5. God gave me asthma because of my past sins.

Reviewing these lists is not supposed to provide you with earth-shattering revelations, but you might get a few surprises. Perhaps you feel angry more often than you used to, but you never connected that feeling with your belief that you, your parents, or your god is to blame for your having asthma. Maybe you think you're just being practical when you decide to stay close to home and avoid vacations and other trips, but if you think about it, you'll realize you've been losing sleep conjuring up catastrophic scenarios about leaving home. Will any insights you get from this review change how you feel? Not automatically, but understanding that some beliefs you hold are based on personalizing events, exaggerating real situations, or that catastrophizing about your life is a step toward reorienting your thinking and in turn keeping emotional reactions appropriate to your true circumstances will help. Following is a simple self-help method that works for many of our asthma patients.

GETTING RID OF FAULTY BELIEFS

None of us walk around knowing that we hold faulty beliefs that make us sad, worried, or angry. In fact, sometimes it's hard for us to realize we're experiencing distressing and uncomfortable feelings. So how do you begin the process of ridding yourself of unrealistic beliefs? Usually, a family member will tell you that something seems wrong and express the desire to help. You should view such an offer as an opportunity to try to understand how you may be feeling and how you can feel better. Lynne used to work as an accountant but now stays at home raising her two preschool-age daughters. She was diagnosed with asthma one year ago and describes how hard it is to keep up with them:

> ‏‏"I'll tell you, I never worked as hard as an accountant as I'm working now with my two girls. Even tax season was a breeze compared to these two. They sure are active, running around the house, climbing on the furniture, bouncing from one activity to the next. It's hard to keep up with them. And sometimes I just can't do it. I get out of breath running after them in the backyard. We

used to play a lot back there, but I just can't do it. I feel terrible about it, because I'm not being a good mother. I'm at home now to play with them, to teach them, to build a family with them, but I'm so limited I sometimes just sit on a chair and cry. I didn't give up my career to be a bad mother. That's not what I want. But that's what it's become. And the girls, well, every time I have to say no, it hurts me, and I think it hurts them too. I don't want them to remember me as the mother who couldn't do anything."

Luckily, Lynne's husband noticed how sad and tearful she was. After John repeatedly approached Lynne, they began to talk about what was troubling her. As they talked, they filled in the following questionnaire, which identifies and then refutes faulty beliefs:

1. What beliefs are bothering you? Lynne and John identified two recurring beliefs that were terribly distressing to Lynne. First, Lynne was a bad mother because she could not play with their children. Second, their daughters did not love her because she could not play with them.

2. What evidence supports these beliefs? Because they were her beliefs, only Lynne could answer this question. She explained that she had stopped working to raise the children and she needed to meet all of their needs. If she could not play with them, she was a bad mother. And children do not love bad mothers. John pointed out that Lynne's answer described her own expectations; it did not provide concrete evidence that she was either a bad or an unloved mother. Lynne then responded that good mothers play with their children all the time, another irrational belief.

3. What evidence refutes these beliefs? John refuted Lynne's two beliefs, with which he strongly disagreed. First, he said that being a good mother is not dependent on any one activity—in Lynne's case, being able to play with the children—but it is multidimensional. He then listed the many things she does for the children, including reading a book to them each evening, sewing new clothes, preparing special meals, and comforting them when they are sick or hurt. He summarized his argument by saying that no one has captured precisely what it means to be a good mother, but all mothers have strengths and weaknesses, and those weaknesses do not necessarily make them bad mothers. To refute her second belief, John brought their two daughters into the room. When they leaped to Lynne and hugged and kissed her, John thought no further evidence was necessary.

4. What would happen if you continued to think this way? Lynne and John agreed that if Lynne continued to think this way she would become more sad and despairing. Her depression could result in less energy and interest in the children, bringing about what she feared most, a withdrawn and ineffective mother.

Lynne and John talked frequently about these beliefs and the evidence; you can't get rid of faulty beliefs during just one conversation. They continued to talk about her beliefs by repeatedly reviewing the four questions listed on the questionnaire. Not only did these talks continue to provide evidence that Lynne's beliefs were faulty, but also Lynne found herself able to talk freely with John about her sadness, anxiety, and asthma. As a result, she felt both supported and understood by her husband. Examining her irrational beliefs, feeling supported by her husband, and mothering her children in other ways eventually made Lynne's depression and tearfulness subside. As her mood improved, Lynne discovered that she had more energy, and she then did even more with her daughters, although running around the backyard was still hard.

Todd's reaction to his asthma was quite different from Lynne's. Todd was angry and resentful at being diagnosed with asthma, and his anger was easy to see:

೭ "I'm not an old man. I'm seventeen years old, and my whole life is ahead of me. I'm not going to let something stupid like asthma keep me from doing the things I want to. I ski, swim, play tennis, and climb mountains, and I don't really care about my asthma. Let me worry about my health when I'm an old guy, not now. I'm young, and young people like me don't have asthma attacks."

Todd saw asthma as a threat to his youthful vitality and active outdoor lifestyle. But after two emergency room visits for asthma exacerbations, Todd's grandfather, Jack, decided to confront him. Jack was also an asthma patient, and he understood well what it meant to live with it. He worried that one day Todd would have an asthma attack far away from a physician or an emergency room. Todd and Jack filled in the questionnaire to refute faulty beliefs:

1. What beliefs are bothering you? Todd stated that nothing was bothering him, that he was doing fine. In contrast, Jack said that Todd seemed angry and bitter about his asthma diagnosis. Jack thought that Todd held the irrational belief that young people do not have asthma. At times this belief was also reflected in the idea that Todd would never have an asthma attack. Because Todd had spoken these words repeatedly, he grudgingly agreed with Jack about the beliefs but denied that he was angry.

2. What evidence supports these beliefs? Because Todd insisted that young people do not have asthma, Jack suggested that he answer this question. Unfortunately, Todd had not read much on asthma; he was always too busy to educate himself about the illness. So he had little evidence to support his belief. Todd just said again that it was his opinion that young people do not have asthma.

3. What evidence refutes these beliefs? Jack decided that simply talking to Todd would not be enough, so he provided him with two very different kinds of evidence. First, Jack showed him an article explaining how asthma afflicts twenty percent of children in the industrialized world, making it the most common chronic disease. And although the death rate among children is relatively low, it is the number-one cause of school absenteeism in the United States. Second, Jack took Todd to a respiratory medicine specialty hospital so he could see for himself what would happen if he did not take care of his asthma. Todd was scared and surprised when he saw the ward devoted solely to adolescents like himself. He talked with several patients who, also like him, had believed that young people could not get asthma.

4. What would happen if you continued to think this way? After Todd visited the hospital, he realized that continuing to think that young people don't get asthma would likely result in more asthma attacks and frequent emergency room visits. As Todd thought about it, he realized that continuing to hold his faulty belief would bring about the outcome he least desired, more reminders that he had asthma.

Jack and Todd continued to talk about their asthma. Todd finally understood how angry he was about his illness, that it made him feel weak and vulnerable and, consequently, he denied its existence. Once he realized what might happen if he continued to avoid his asthma, he became more interested in learning about his illness and how he could best manage it. He was relieved to discover that, with proper management, he could continue the physical activities he so enjoyed.

In many respects, Todd's attitude is similar to that of Cindy, who was described in Chapter 2. Both wanted to keep their asthma from affecting their active life and tried to continue participating in sports. However, this denial of asthma had different sources for Todd and Cindy. Todd's denial was fueled by his anger and rage at having asthma. His sport activities were just another expression of his anger. Cindy's denial was fueled by her need to maintain her healthy, active body image. Anger, anxiety, or sadness were not as apparent as her fixation on body image. So, just as people like Eddie and Todd can have vastly different emotional reactions to asthma, individuals can have similar responses (such as denial and noncompliance with medical advice) for different reasons. If you're having trouble living well with asthma, only you can determine with certainty what is going on in your mind and heart.

Identifying faulty beliefs is hard work and requires unflinching honesty. It starts with listening to the important people around you. They want you to live a full, productive life and would not confront you with their observations if they were not concerned. So listen to those who care about you. They can help you identify and modify faulty beliefs that might be causing you distress.

MAKING PEACE WITH ASTHMA

None of this discussion about identifying faulty beliefs means you should expect your life to be a paradigm of serenity. You *will* have reactions to living with asthma. If you didn't think so, you wouldn't be reading this book. Sadness, anger, panic, and apathy are all important parts of asthma. For most people these reactions, although at times strong, do not become debilitating. Yet you cannot always address them by yourself. Frequently, someone else is necessary to help you look objectively and realistically at what you're feeling and the faulty beliefs that may be responsible for the distressing emotion. Don't go it alone! There are always people around who care about you and want to help. Take advantage of their interest and concern. Inevitably, something will arise in their lives and they will need *your* help. (Yes, even people without asthma sometimes need assistance and support.) If the two of you working together cannot get a handle on your feelings, and they are distressing or debilitating, see a professional. Living with asthma is challenging, but living with asthma while depressed, anxious, or enraged is unnecessarily difficult. Here are a few more suggestions for dealing with your feelings.

Staying Calm by Staying Informed

Nobody likes feeling anxious. It's scary experiencing the panic, shortness of breath, and pounding heart that accompany an anxiety attack. In many respects, an asthma exacerbation has similar symptoms, and for some people, including doctors, it's difficult to distinguish between the two. However, one thing is certain: an asthma attack makes anyone feel nervous. You're frightened that the next gasp of air will be your last! Unfortunately, it also appears that anxiety makes breathing worse during an asthma attack, making it important to stay calm. But how? The panic, helplessness, and breathing problems are overwhelming! Well, probably the best way to control your anxiety is to educate yourself about your asthma. Talk to your doctor. Read books like this one. Do peak flow metering so you know when you're beginning to get into trouble and can stop it before it becomes a problem. Learn what to do when you start to have symptoms of an asthma attack to better control it; here, too, your doctor and any of the books available on the medical aspects of asthma can help. Education is the key to curbing panic. Knowing what to do and diverting your attention to doing it short-circuits anxiety and allows you to keep your cool.

Finding a Physical Release

Being depressed, angry, or anxious is draining, even exhausting. It may not feel like hard work, but it robs you of energy that you made no conscious decision to expend. Actively channeling your finite energy supplies into some physical form of release offers numerous benefits, not the least of which is relieving stress, thereby reducing depression, anger, and anxiety before they can sap your strength. Swimming, walking, or just about any physical activity can help you feel better because, for example, exercise produces chemicals in the brain that will make you feel happier and more content. Regular exercise can also create a sense of accomplishment and empowerment. Knowing that you're using your energy to better your health rather than passively accepting the exhaustion of chronic sadness and fear increases your self-esteem and insulates you from depression. When you're angry, sad, or nervous, exercise can distract you from the thoughts (remember, the *thoughts*, not the events) that lead to distressing feelings. After exercising you can review these faulty beliefs more calmly and objectively. Finally, exercising helps you feel better about your body despite the asthma. So, don't just sit here reading this book. Take a moment to think of an exercise you can begin and enjoy today.

Rejecting the Medication Scapegoat

Again, when you're feeling downhearted it's often tough to delve into your beliefs to get at the root of your feelings. Sometimes it just seems easier to go back to blaming events themselves. A popular scapegoat in such cases is medication. Although it may be convenient to blame your sadness, anxiety, or anger on your medications, the truth is that they are usually not responsible for how you feel. Oral steroids can affect your mood, but not very severely or consistently. If you're beginning steroid treatment, you may find yourself feeling slightly elated and excited. You may act overly cheerful, energetic, and happy. With prolonged steroid use, your mood can swing between this happiness and elation and mild sadness, as if you're on a gentle roller coaster. The best way to get off this roller coaster is to stay on as low a dosage of steroids as possible. You may also notice that you experience mood changes when treated with a sudden burst of high-dosage steroids yet feel fine when on your usual oral steroid level. Mood shifts of more than mild severity likely have other causes. If you have any concerns about your medication and your mood, talk to your doctor. Once you've ruled out medications as a cause, you can turn back to the methods in this chapter for getting rid of faulty beliefs and assuaging negative emotions.

✃ Chapter 4

"I Use My Inhaler in the Bathroom."

As we've just seen, faulty or irrational beliefs about asthma can lead to unnecessary sadness, anxiety, fear, or anger. These exaggerated emotional responses don't just make people uncomfortable, however. They also alter behavior. Lynne's distress over feeling inadequate as a mother caused her to spend increasingly less time with her daughters, precisely the opposite of what she truly wanted. Todd's anger over having to acknowledge his asthma at the age of seventeen pushed him to pursue his beloved sports with a vengeance, which only ended up reminding him of his condition. Unresolved emotion based on faulty beliefs can make one of the greatest fears about asthma—that it will change *you* irrevocably—a self-fulfilling prophecy: you begin to act like someone else. Over the course of your life with asthma, if you catch yourself wondering why you're behaving the way you are (or when others begin to point out that "you don't seem to be yourself"), it's time to reexamine your beliefs as laid out in Chapter 3. You may find you're operating on a new, faulty belief about asthma.

This chapter addresses one particular area of behavior that is impacted greatly by your beliefs: how you follow medical advice, especially the use of asthma medications. Marty's experience illustrates how psychological factors can affect the medical management of asthma and how poor medical management can in turn have psychological and social consequences.

&ewline; Marty is a forty-four-year-old senior account executive with a well-known insurance company, and she has asthma. She has worked with the same company for eighteen years, advancing from secretary to senior account executive. She has done very well in a male-dominated field through what she describes as a combination of "smarts and toughness." It is Marty's belief that any signs of weakness regarding her commitment to the job, ability to work long hours, or any physical problems would spell the end of her rise through the firm.

    Marty's doctor prescribes that she take inhaled treatments four times a day, two of them during work hours. Marty usually waits until no one is present in the rest room, then uses her inhaler in a bathroom stall. When the timing is not convenient, she skips the treatment altogether, something that happens about one-third of the time. As Marty puts it, "I'm not embarrassed by my inhaler, but I know enough about the glass ceiling to keep my health problems to myself. I don't want to give them any reasons to question my ability to work side by side with the men in the office."

Eventually Marty did run into problems because of her asthma, but not the kind she had imagined. Although her co-workers did not know she had asthma, they had noticed her regular trips to the rest room. Rumors had started about Marty, ranging from "emotional problems" to "female health problems," and even to the possibility that she was using street drugs at work. When her boss confronted her with the rumors, noting that she did sometimes appear "hyper" after using the rest room, Marty explained what she was doing and why. She had asthma, was using prescribed medications as ordered, and, yes, she did occasionally get a little jittery after a treatment.

    Marty's boss was greatly relieved to hear the news. After all, she was a valued, hardworking employee, and the rumors about her had seemed out of character. As it turned out, her boss's son also had asthma, as did two men that he knew of in the office. He assured her not only that her having asthma would in no way change his thinking about her, but also that he would deal with anyone who did treat her poorly. Marty was now free to use her inhaler whenever and wherever she wanted, and her sense of relief was enormous. Interestingly, some of the jitteriness that she had believed was a medication side effect also disappeared, because Marty was no longer looking over her shoulder, trying to hide a normal part of her life. The only job impact her openness seemed to have was the new respect her co-workers showed when she explained what had been occurring.

Marty had held a faulty belief that her standing in the company would diminish if it was known that she had asthma. The evidence for this belief came not from direct observation but from an assumption about what it took for a woman to be successful in her industry. The assumption was that asthma would be viewed by others as a sign of weakness and that she would not be treated fairly by her peers and her boss. Again, this was not based on direct evidence, but she nevertheless believed strongly that it was true. If she had continued to think this way, her health would surely have suffered, and her reputation would likely have suffered as well. Ironically, what Marty wanted to avoid (others viewing her as being weak) was exactly what was beginning to evolve.

The opposite turned out to be true. When Marty confided in her boss, he provided all the evidence she needed to refute her faulty belief, and the subsequent behavior of her co-workers provided further support. As a result of refuting that belief, Marty changed the way she cared for herself, and her asthma improved.

For Marty, the concern that led to rejecting her own care was not wanting to appear weak to her co-workers. For Bill it was even more complicated.

&ep; Bill refused to follow any of his doctor's recommendations. He did not really know why, but he knew that he felt "like a child" whenever he took medications of any type. As the owner of a small restaurant, Bill wanted to feel like an adult. His responsibilities were certainly adult. As a young boy, Bill had had asthma, and like many children with asthma, he had been teased by his friends for needing to use an inhaler and for not being able to participate in sports. Even though he had been a big kid, he had been called a "sissy" more times than he wished to remember. One of Bill's most painful memories from childhood was not being allowed to go to summer camp with his friends. The camp was on a dusty ranch in Montana, and Bill's parents thought he would have too much trouble breathing in that environment. After this embarrassment he was also called a "mama's boy" by some of the unkindest children.

Bill longed to be anything but a mama's boy. As he matured he became more and more independent, not only of his asthma, which had improved dramatically during his twenties, but in all aspects of his life. He was a hard worker and an independent thinker. After college he was offered a number of jobs in the hotel/restaurant industry, but Bill did not want to work for anyone else. He preferred to be his own boss, to be independent. And he was successful.

When Bill's asthma began to worsen again in his early thirties, he initially refused to see a doctor. Even after he did see an allergist for one appointment, Bill steadfastly refused to use the oral medications and inhalers that were prescribed. Predictably, Bill's asthma got worse, not better.

Bill was making a mistake that most of us make at one time or another: he was trying to avoid painful feelings from his past by neglecting parts of his present life. Bill's childhood had been painful, especially regarding how he had been treated about his asthma. Now that his asthma was back, he wished to avoid all the bad feelings that went with being called "sissy" and "mama's boy." After all, that did not fit his image of himself as an independent entrepreneur. What he didn't realize was that to get rid of those old, painful feelings, he had to face them as an adult, not avoid them. Facing them meant acknowledging them, understanding where they came from, and realizing that, in the present, things could be very different.

Eventually Bill's asthma got so bad that it began to interfere with work. He avoided the restaurant first thing in the morning because the smell of cleaning fluids was too strong, and he had trouble breathing in the hot, congested kitchen. Ironically, some of the early-morning employees began to talk about him as "too lazy" to come in early, comments that would have reminded Bill of names he had been called as a child.

One night Bill went to the emergency room because his breathing was so bad. While waiting to see a doctor, a rather blunt nurse listened to his story and said, "I know your problem. You're too much of a baby to take your medicine." This seemed all wrong to Bill, and it made him angry. He didn't want to be like a child. That was why he *didn't* take his medication, wasn't it? As a child, Bill's asthma had caused him social embarrassment, and he believed that if it had not been for his asthma he would not have felt so humiliated. This was, unfortunately, a correct belief based on an accurate picture of his childhood. However, as an adult, Bill had never reexamined that belief, and it was no longer true. What had been accurate when he was a child had turned into a faulty belief when he became an adult. As a child, asthma had made him feel weak and dependent; as an adult, *ignoring* his asthma had made him weak and dependent.

Sitting there in the emergency room, it dawned on Bill just how much he hated the role that asthma had played in his life. He began to realize that the nurse was right. The evidence was clear that in his attempt to avoid feeling like a child, he was acting like one. If he continued to think and act this way his asthma would get worse, and he would feel more child-like, dependent, and miserable. Right there and then, Bill decided to change. He was an adult, and if that meant taking medications, he could do that. In fact, he told himself, "Every time I take my asthma medications, it makes me more of an independent adult." His new belief was accurate. For a few weeks he used that saying every day to help him take his medications. Within a month Bill no longer needed the saying. Besides, he was too busy at work.

Trouble taking care of your asthma is likely a problem of faulty beliefs, not a wish to harm yourself, thwart your doctor, or limit your ability to function in daily life. Marty believed that if she used her inhaler publicly, others would think her weak.

This was a faulty belief about her company, based on a series of observations that had some truth (women needed to be hard-working) but were incorrect regarding her asthma. Until she was forced to check it out, however, how could she discover she was wrong? Bill believed that taking medications would make him feel as he had as a child. The opposite turned out to be more accurate; that is, when he took control of his asthma, he felt more adult; when he avoided his medications, his asthma worsened, and he felt and acted more like a child. Sally had a different sort of faulty belief about herself and her asthma.

> When Sally looked at her inhaler, she cringed. A pretty, twenty-nine-year-old woman, Sally told herself and her friends that she was very interested in being in a committed relationship with a man. But she didn't believe any man could truly like her because she was so limited by her asthma and the need for medications and inhaled treatments. What must others think of her and her silly inhaler? How could anyone like her, find her attractive? At times Sally felt quite lonely, and she blamed her asthma.
>
> When Sally met Tom, she liked him right away. And, at first, Tom seemed to like her too. On their third date, however, Sally needed to use her inhaler in the movie theater, and she thought she noticed that Tom looked away while she did. "There he goes," thought Sally, "another man who turns away from me when he sees I have asthma." Sally was so hurt and angry that the rest of the night was a disaster. Because she was angry she was cold toward Tom; because she felt hurt she withdrew from him person-ally and physically. Although they dated a few more times, the initial spark never returned, and Sally was left once again looking for a relationship with a man who could tolerate her asthma.

Sally believed that others would find her unattractive if they saw her use her inhaler, so she acted sensibly based on that faulty belief. When Sally believed that a man found her unat-tractive, she became disinterested in him. After all, why try to have a romantic relationship with someone who finds you unattractive? However, Sally's belief was faulty. Other people did not really find Sally unattractive when she used her inhaler. The truth was that Sally found *herself* unattractive when she used her inhaler.

Unfortunately, Sally was not aware of this, and so she

tended to experience other people as "turned off" by her asthma. Until she could recognize this about herself, she was at risk to repeat the pattern over and over with the men she dated. This can be a serious problem with faulty beliefs; once you have one you tend to keep it until you have enough evidence to refute it. That is what happened to Sally. She dated a number of men but never seemed to get beyond the fifth or sixth date before she began to believe that the men "couldn't handle" her asthma. It was Sally's therapist who finally helped Sally challenge and refute her faulty beliefs.

Sally decided to see a therapist because of her unhappiness regarding men. In the first session she told her therapist that she was angry at men in general because they seemed to expect her to be perfect, especially regarding her health. Every time a man saw she had asthma, he withdrew.

Sally and her therapist stayed focused on this topic for most of their ten sessions. By the third session the therapist had correctly challenged Sally's faulty belief that it was men who could not tolerate her asthma. Over the next few sessions Sally and her therapist found much evidence to refute this idea, and by the time they ended Sally was at least willing to approach her next date a little differently, and see if she was being oversensitive to how men were responding to her asthma. Once Sally was aware that it was *she*, not men she dated, who "couldn't handle" her asthma, she was in a much better position to meet men and consider a serious relationship. She was even able to reexamine her time with Tom and realize that Tom's turning away was probably not a sign that she was unattractive but his attempt to help her avoid possible embarrassment.

Sally had been unaware of not only her own feelings of unattractiveness regarding her asthma but also her own nervousness about being in a committed relationship. Although Sally told herself and her friends that she wanted a relationship, the truth was that on a deep level she was not so sure. She wanted a relationship but was also fearful that if she had one she might not be happy, or it might end in divorce.

Sally blamed her asthma and men's reactions to it for her difficulty keeping a relationship going. Actually Sally, not her asthma, was preventing her from having a committed relationship. Without even knowing it, Sally was using her asthma as an excuse. Her therapy allowed her to refute her faulty beliefs and begin to confront her real fears of relationships, this time without any excuses.

STEP 1 TOWARD SUCCESSFUL MEDICAL MANAGEMENT: KNOW WHEN TO REVIEW YOUR BELIEFS

Bill, Marty, and Sally all relied on important others to help them notice and refute their faulty beliefs. It is true that other people who care about you can be an important source of information and support. Resist the temptation to see them as simply nagging or nosy.

But you needn't rely just upon others. *The simple fact that you receive medical advice that you are not following should be a red flag that faulty beliefs may be at work.* Before you decide to ignore or deviate from the advice of medical professionals, ask yourself if faulty beliefs might be guiding you. If they are, what might those beliefs be? What is the evidence that supports or might refute those beliefs? Use the questionnaire in Chapter 3 as a means of imposing checks and balances on yourself and your health care team. No one is infallible, but always remember that you have final veto power for a reason: Ultimately, you do know what is best for you; after all, *it is your asthma.* Your decision to deviate from medical advice may prove to be based on sound, rational thinking, as it was for Elinor.

  Elinor is a thirty-eight-year-old librarian who has had mild asthma since she was a young girl. In the last three or four years, however, her asthma has worsened, so she reluctantly went to a pulmonologist to "get it under control." The doctor recommended that Elinor begin taking regular, inhaled medication three times a day and oral medication twice a day, change her diet, and begin regular exercise so she could lose twenty-five pounds, as well as avoid certain environments such as dusty rooms.

    When Elinor returned for her next appointment three weeks

later, she was happy to report that she had used the medication as prescribed and was feeling much better. She was surprised to find that her doctor, rather than being glad for her, was angry that she had not been on a diet, had not started regular exercise, and had not switched to a less dusty part of the library. He used the term *noncompliant*. "Whose asthma is this?" Elinor wondered.

It is your asthma. Not your family's, your friends', your boss's, your therapist's, or even your doctor's. Elinor's doctor wrote in her chart that she took her prescribed medications but was noncompliant with the remainder of her program. Elinor, on the other hand, felt that she had done a good job of arranging her schedule so that she could take all the medications and inhaled treatments as ordered, and she was happy with the results. This scenario points out an essential feature of medical self-care: compliance is in the eye of the beholder.

Elinor believed that some of her doctor's recommendations were more important to her than others. Her evidence for this was quite good; when she followed the recommendations she thought most important, for example, taking her medications as prescribed, she felt better. She believed that her asthma would improve if she used the proper medications, so she acted on that belief. Elinor's belief was correct; she did feel much better.

Elinor also believed that losing twenty-five pounds would require an effort she was not prepared to give at that time. She had tried dieting several times in the past and believed that dieting did not work for long. To permanently lower her weight would require a lifestyle change, not a diet. Elinor was not ready to make that lifestyle change and believed, correctly, that she should not attempt a major weight loss until she was truly ready.

Similarly, Elinor was not ready to change jobs at the library. Although a move to the cleaner computer room was possible, she perceived that people who worked there did not move easily up the library stepladder. She believed, correctly, that such a change would limit her opportunities for advancement. In other words, the change might be good for her asthma, but it would be bad for her. Elinor acted reasonably on her correct beliefs. She did not request a job change as recommended by her doctor.

She also carefully examined all of these beliefs using the process described in Chapter 3 and asked friends as well what they thought of her decisions. Her beliefs held up to this scrutiny: The improvement she observed in her breathing when she took medications bore out her belief that medication was important. Her knowledge of herself supported her belief that lifestyle changes required more effort than she was presently prepared to give.

STEP 2 TOWARD SUCCESSFUL MEDICAL MANAGEMENT: ACT ON ACCURATE BELIEFS

In the end, Elinor acted on her own accurate beliefs rather than strictly on her doctor's orders. She took her medication but did not go on a diet or begin an exercise program. Despite her doctor's statement that she was noncompliant, Elinor felt much better physically and much happier. Elinor's experience underscores how important it is, once you have confirmed the accuracy of your beliefs, that you trust yourself and act on them.

Once you have checked the validity of your beliefs, let them lead you to a course of action. ACT ON YOUR BELIEFS! If you believe medication makes you feel better, take medication. If good self-care makes you feel like a competent adult, take good care of yourself. If you believe some things are good for you but others are not, do the things you truly believe are in your best interests. Remember, an accurate belief that you do not act on is no better than having no accurate beliefs at all.

A MEDICAL MANAGEMENT TRIPLE THREAT

The stories of Marty, Bill, Sally, and Elinor illustrate three beliefs that most commonly stand as obstacles to good medical self-management. All three are patently false, yet they can be difficult to topple because they typically spring from deeply held fears of isolation, failure, and abandonment. If you find yourself rejecting medical advice, reviewing the following list in tandem with using the questionnaire in Chapter 3 may help you ascertain that any medical actions you take from now on are based only on valid beliefs.

1. *"People will think of me as weak if they know I have asthma."* This belief may lead you to hide your asthma from others at work, socially, or with family. Hiding your asthma will likely mean hiding the treatment of your asthma as well, leaving you at risk for less than optimal self-care. An important component of this belief is that *you* may be one of the people who will view you as weak if you have asthma! Examine the validity of these beliefs carefully.

It is true that a few people uneducated about asthma may view you as weak or that you may view yourself as weak or inadequate because of your asthma. For the majority of people, however, this belief is inaccurate. Prove it to yourself by beginning to reveal your asthma gradually. Start with those that you don't perceive as having too much power over you (not those who hold your job security in their hands); they undoubtedly will give you the confidence to be open with everyone.

2. *"People will not like me if I have asthma."* Again, it may be that some people truly will not like you or find you attractive because of your asthma. For most people, however, this belief turns out to be false. Be sure that other people are not simply uncomfortable around you because they do not know how to act. If that is the case, tell them *how* you would like them to act. Most important, be sure that it is not you that finds your asthma unattractive, even though you experience the dislike as coming from other people. Become aware of how you feel about your asthma as a way of checking your beliefs about how you think other people feel about your asthma.

3. *"If I don't do everything my doctor recommends, I won't get the best treatment."* As we discuss in Chapter 11, your doctor is an expert consultant. Only you, however, can ultimately decide what is best for you. That does not mean you take the easy way out, follow only those recommendations that are easy, and

ignore the rest. Be honest with yourself. Carefully and honestly examine the reasons for your self-care decisions. If your reasons for refusing to follow certain advice prove valid, don't be cowed by the term *noncompliant,* typically used by doctors to describe patients who do not do everything the doctor tells them to do. The nurse in the emergency room accused Bill of noncompliance, and Marty's doctor may have described her as noncompliant for using her inhaler only when no one could see her do so. Unfortunately, patients who are called noncompliant may feel blamed by their doctor, with the implication that if they do not follow orders, they deserve what they get. Therefore, *noncompliant* has become something of a dirty word to patients caught in a battle of wills with their physician, and sometimes that battle becomes so intense that patients refuse to follow their doctors' orders as a way of striking out and asserting their own will over the doctor's. Obviously, everyone loses in this case, but especially the patient. If you fear that resentment is building between you and your doctor over who is the authority in your relationship, try to discuss the issue with him or her; some suggestions are given in Chapter 11. If you can't resolve the problem, you may be better off finding another doctor. Remember, *act on your beliefs—as long as they are accurate!*

Chapter 5

"My Normal Lifestyle Isn't Over After All—I'm Stronger and Happier Than Ever!"

Change, even when welcome, is unsettling. Unsolicited change, such as the initial diagnosis of asthma or the return of a disease you had hoped was behind you, can knock you right off your feet.

How do you typically respond to uninvited change in your life? How have you been reacting to the diagnosis or recurrence of asthma so far? You've seen how some people respond to specific issues that usually arise with asthma—altered body image, troublesome emotions, and compliance with medical advice—and now know where some of your own sticking points may lie. But if what you've learned so far hasn't been enough to help you live well with asthma, rest assured that no one adapts to chronic illness overnight. We all have our own characteristic ways of responding to life's unwanted surprises, and sometimes our initial response to the diagnosis of asthma can stand in the way of a thoroughly successful adaptation to life with this disease. Understanding your own responses, combined with use of the self-check techniques provided in Chapters 2–4, should help you get back on your feet and on the road to living well with asthma.

Any journey is easier to undertake when it's broken down into manageable stretches, so try to view this trip as having three legs: diagnosis, response, and adaptation. If you're reading this book, you've already finished the first leg, which puts you well on your way to your destination. Bob and Margaret are just setting out.

DIAGNOSIS: A TIME OF UNCERTAINTY

&> It started for Bob at a cocktail party one night when his host, who happened to be an internist, asked, "Are you wheezing?" "No, I'm not wheezing," Bob immediately replied, although he felt a little unsure about exactly what wheezing was. He had been noticing lately that when he exerted himself, he had a little trouble catching his breath. But he figured that was what being forty years old meant: harder to stay in shape, harder to catch your breath, and all of that—but not wheezing. Wheezing was something for old people with oxygen tanks, wasn't it?

At his company's health fair several weeks later, Bob asked the nurse who was having people blow into a tube if he was wheezing. She confirmed that he was, suggested it might be undiagnosed asthma, and recommended he schedule an appointment with his family doctor. Bob's first response was "Well, that can't be right," and he did not schedule the recommended appointment.

&> Margaret generally skipped the evening news, because all it seemed to contain were horror stories about airline crashes, crimes, and rising interest rates. She generally considered herself a lucky person, an optimist, and watching one bad story after another made her feel nervous. Margaret was also just a little bit superstitious and thought it was best to stay away from the unpleasant parts of life as much as possible. And Margaret was lucky. She was twenty-nine, happily married to the supervisor of electricians for a large construction company, and this allowed her to stay at home and care for their two young girls, ages six and four. Except for the fact that she and her husband had wanted a boy and a girl, things had worked out pretty well so far. Knock on wood.

Margaret took pretty good care of herself, watched her diet, went for walks, and with the two girls around, she tended to stay quite active. Still, like many others, she had caught the flu last winter, and when most of the symptoms were gone, a cough and strange tightness in her chest remained. Not one to stick her head in the sand, Margaret went to her doctor, who diagnosed asthma.

Margaret fully intended to do everything the doctor recommended—get some further testing, begin inhaled treatments—but for some reason she became so preoccupied with her daughters' health that she forgot about her own. It seemed that since her diagnosis of asthma, the girls were getting more runny noses and spring coughs than usual. Despite her pediatrician's assessment that the girls' colds were nothing out of the ordinary, Margaret began to worry that they might have developed allergies and started investigating how to get them tested. "I guess you can't avoid all of life's troubles," she lamented to herself, but she was determined to do whatever was necessary to get the girls healthy again. Then, she would have time to focus on her asthma.

When you were first told you had asthma, you probably knew little about what that meant. Unless you had a family member or close friend with asthma, your knowledge of the illness was likely quite limited. Maybe you had heard that some Olympic athletes had asthma but had overcome it. Possibly you'd seen a recent news story about asthma being on the rise in inner-city neighborhoods. Or you may have been familiar with one of the common myths about asthma discussed in Chapter 1. For example, you may have heard that asthma is all in your head. Whatever accurate information about this respiratory disease you possessed, it undoubtedly wasn't enough to satisfy you upon your diagnosis.

Uncertainty is the hallmark of the diagnostic phase of asthma. What does *asthma* mean? How did I get it? Why did I get it? What should I do? How will my life be changed? What kind of doctor will I need to see? Will it be expensive to treat? How long will it last? Does this mean my children will get it too? These and many other questions probably started to tumble through your mind the moment your name and asthma were linked. Then, along came fear and apprehension, uncertainty's constant companions.

Though many people try to hide it out of misguided shame, fear is almost guaranteed to be the dominant emotion during the diagnostic phase of asthma. It's only human nature; when we are unsure about something important that impacts us directly, we often respond with some degree of fear. That does not make you a coward. Responding to uncertainty with fear has been part of the human condition for as long as we know. In fact, the link between uncertainty and fear is part of our evolutionary heritage; it is a natural response that has helped assure the survival of our species. Early on, human beings learned that when faced with something new and unsettling, it's best not to stick your neck out too far. Better to pull back a little, regroup, and learn more about the situation. Then, adapt in as healthy a way as possible.

There are two ways to handle the fear of the diagnostic phase: (1) accept it; (2) resolve as much of your uncertainty as you can. Not taking these measures, in fact, is a sure way to stall your progress toward adaptation. You can't hope to resolve your fear if you don't admit it's there, and you can't assuage your fear if you don't resolve the uncertainty that is causing it. Whenever you feel anxious about your diagnosis, remind yourself that your fear is only natural and that it will pass. If it helps, talk to someone about it. Meanwhile, get all the information you can. Keep a running list of all the questions you want to ask your doctor, and start tapping the information resources available to you (see the Appendix at the end of this book).

RESPONSE: YOUR PSYCHOLOGICAL DEFENSES

Beyond the uncertainty and fear that accompany diagnosis, you likely responded to the news in ways that were fairly typical for you. When faced with something new and unsettling, like a medical diagnosis, we tend to respond in our own characteristic ways. These first, characteristic ways of responding are sometimes called our *psychological defenses*. Understanding your defenses and how they contribute to your response to the diagnosis of asthma can be a key to helping you adapt to your asthma in healthy, productive ways.

Even if your responses to diagnosis do not seem to be serving you particularly well, don't get the idea that psychological defenses are all bad. These defenses are one important way the human mind copes with fear and uncertainty. Without them, you would easily become overwhelmed by life's uncertainties and unpleasant events, and you would feel too afraid to think, plan, and adapt. Defenses are an important way we pull back and give ourselves the time and opportunity to learn more. They allow us to catch our breath before facing a new challenge, something important for all of us, especially asthma patients. So, defenses are necessary and useful. However, they can also be too much of a good thing. When your natural defenses get in the way of your making good choices about your asthma, they can cause problems. Bob and Margaret, for example, illustrate two of the most common defenses to the diagnosis of asthma, the twin D's of denial and displacement.

Denial

Bob tends to deny that bad things have happened to him. This is his usual response to potentially bad news. The bigger the news, the more he uses the psychological defense of denial. This means that rather than feel the fear of uncertainty that follows the diagnosis of asthma, he pretends to others and even to himself that he doesn't have asthma at all. "Well, that can't be right," Bob concludes about the diagnosis, and he decides not to see his doctor for an initial visit. Bob's defense is so strong that it has become too much of a good thing. Yes, his denial is keeping away his fear, but it is also keeping Bob out of his doctor's office, where he could begin to get information that is truly necessary to help reduce his uncertainty and his fear.

Displacement

Margaret doesn't deny that she has asthma, but she has become much more concerned about her girls' health than her own. This is the defense of displacement, when our fears are shifted from ourselves to someone else. In this example, Margaret may be concerned about her asthma, but she focuses her time and attention on her children's health instead. This is Margaret's way of not focusing on her own fear of uncertainty. Displacement is a favorite defense of very caring people, people who are more at ease taking care of others than themselves. Like Bob, Margaret's first response to the diagnosis of asthma has come between herself and the care she needs. Margaret's use of displacement is causing her to put off a needed visit to the doctor. She says that she'll go when her girls are healthy. When do you think that might be?

Intellectualization

Another common defense that you may use after learning you have asthma is intellectualization, also known as the thinking defense. This is a common defense with people who are more comfortable with their intellect than their feelings, who usually use their intellect to help lessen their fears. Troy, a young family law attorney, uses this defense, but not to the extent that it causes him much trouble. It never becomes too much of a good thing.

> ଈ When Troy learned he had asthma, he responded to the news as he would to any new problem that he didn't know enough about: he went straight to the library. This time it wasn't the law library, but the health resources section of his city library that he headed for. He spent the better part of three days in that library, and by the time he came up for air, Troy knew what asthma was, how it was typically treated, and he had decided to consult first his family doctor, then a pulmonologist, if necessary.

Troy's defense of intellectualization led him right into the adaptation phase of coping with his asthma. It led him directly into a mode of learning more, which can be a wonderful cure for the fear of uncertainty. The only place Troy put himself at risk for too much of that good thing was in how he handled his feelings about the new diagnosis. Troy noticed he had almost no feelings at all about his asthma except for the initial fear of uncertainty, which left him soon after his time in the library. This means that in Troy's attempts to learn about his asthma, he also shut out most of his other feelings about the diagnosis, such as sadness or anger.

It is important to have your own feelings about asthma and not shut them out altogether. However, as we said in Chapter 3, while it is normal to have a range of feelings about your asthma, and important to acknowledge them, it is not necessary to let them debilitate you. Facing your feelings about your asthma can also help you identify what faulty beliefs (Chapter 3) might be standing in your way to a healthy adaptation. Nevertheless, if Troy went a little too far, at least he went in the right direction—right to some good sources of information about asthma and then to his physician.

Projection and Rationalization

Denial, displacement, and intellectualization are the most common defenses employed during the response stage of asthma, but other defenses may also be at work. One of these is projection, seeing your feelings as occurring in someone else without knowing you're doing so: "I'm not worried about my asthma diagnosis, but my wife sure is. Maybe she ought to speak to someone about it."

Another defense, similar to Troy's, is rationalization, also used by people who like to use their intellect and stay away from their feelings. Rationalizers might say to themselves, "I read a lot, and I haven't heard much about asthma. If asthma was really such a problem, why haven't I heard more about it? When I hear more about it, maybe I'll take it more seriously and consult with my doctor."

Identifying Your Own Defenses

What is your defensive style? To answer this question, think back to some important and unsettling events in your life, such as changes in your work, your relationships, or your health, and examine your initial reactions. If you are honest with yourself, you may be able to find a pattern or typical way you responded in the various situations. Look especially for the common defenses just described. When life's problems hit, do you tend to deny them at first? Do you get more concerned with other things than the problem at hand? Do you try to think your way out of the event's being a problem at all? Might you project your worry or concerns onto someone else or try to rationalize them away? It is possible that you use a combination of these defenses, but usually you'll be able to spot one dominant defense nonetheless.

If you cannot identify which defense(s) you tend to rely on, ask someone who knows you well. Sometimes it is difficult to see ourselves objectively, and asking someone close to you if he or she has noticed a common way you respond may help get you started. Remember, defenses are not abnormal; we all have them, we all use them, and they are very necessary to our psychological survival. However, overuse can prevent us from moving into the adaptation phase of coping with asthma.

Recognizing the defense(s) you used when you initially learned you had asthma is an important step in allowing you to move into the third stage of the process, adapting to asthma in a healthy, productive way. Bob's denial was preventing him from even being diagnosed; Margaret's displacement was preventing her from getting a full diagnosis and beginning her treatment. Until they acknowledged what they were doing to avoid accepting asthma, neither could hope to control the physical symptoms of asthma, much less lead a liberated, satisfying life. Troy's defense, as we've said, actually moved him forward rather than holding him back. However, unless he acknowledges the feelings he has about asthma, his anger and sadness could build into

future resentment or depression. This means that a little intro-
spection is a wise move on each leg of your journey:

*Anytime you notice persistent, heightened emotions that you can't
explain, use the questionnaire in Chapter 3 to try to trace the beliefs
behind them.*

  ❧ Two years after his initial diagnosis, Troy's asthma was under
control, he was accustomed to a modified lifestyle that suited his
medical needs, and he still read everything he could find on
developments in asthma research and care. Suddenly, though, he
began to notice that he often had a stiff neck, and his girlfriend
started complaining that he seemed increasingly irritable these
days. After ongoing discussions, initiated within the framework of
the questionnaire in Chapter 3, Troy uncovered a belief that he
ultimately saw as faulty: it wasn't okay for him to be angry about
having asthma because, after all, being angry wouldn't change
anything.

    Eventually, Troy couldn't deny the logic of seeking help with
acknowledging his emotions and relieving his stress. His physician
referred him to a therapist, who has taught Troy various stress
management techniques and is available for consultation when
Troy feels he needs to sort out his emotions and his thoughts.

ADAPTATION: FLOURISHING THROUGH INNER STRENGTH

Bob, Margaret, and Troy each responded differently to the diagnosis of asthma, but they all relied on an inner strength that
already existed within them to face the illness and learn to adapt
to it in healthy, productive ways.

When Bob learned he had asthma, he denied it to himself
and to his family. This was not Bob's first encounter with denial;
it was his usual way of responding to upsetting news. In the
past, Bob had shown the ability to get past his denial and move
into more productive ways of coping with life's problems:

  ❧ About five years before he began having problems with asthma,
Bob learned the company he worked for was downsizing. At first,
he denied this, said it couldn't happen to him, and did little about

it. After a couple of weeks, however, Bob noticed that others in the office were taking the rumors much more seriously than he. Not wanting to be left out, Bob set about updating his résumé and sending it to prospective employers. Ultimately, his company did downsize, but a month before the reduction was actually announced, Bob was already working for a new firm. In other words, even though Bob's initial reaction to the rumors was denial, he used the model of how others were responding to help him break through his denial and move into a more adaptive way of coping with the stress of the downsizing. Drawing on this positive experience of getting past his defenses, Bob was able to do something similar with his asthma.

Since the night of that cocktail party, Bob had been having dreams of the time at work when he first denied, then acted on the rumors and landed himself a new job. When he mentioned the dreams to his wife, Laurie, she commented, "Maybe that's because you're sticking your head in the sand with your asthma just like you did back then with your job?" Bob valued and relied on Laurie's insights; sometimes she seemed to know more about him than he did, and this one rang true. That night, Bob dreamed he was updating his résumé again, but this time it was his "health résumé," not his employment history. That was enough for him; between Laurie's comment and his dreams, he knew what to do.

Bob actually did exactly what he had dreamed; he updated his health résumé. He took an honest accounting of his health and lifestyle, then made an appointment for a general medical physical. On the résumé were his many strengths; after all, he was in generally good health. But also on the résumé were some question marks, such as weight, blood pressure, and asthma.

Bob got past his initial, characteristic defense and was now on course for adapting to his asthma. To do so, he relied on several sources for help, including his experience of having gotten past denial at work, his wife's insights about his behavior, and even his own dreams! Interestingly, he then used his asthma as an opportunity to take a more general look at his health and lifestyle, probably a useful approach for a forty-five-year-old man. Rather than stay stuck in denial, Bob became aware of several health items that needed attention, including his diet, weight, blood pressure, and newly diagnosed asthma. It turned out that each of these areas of concern were connected and easier to treat because he attended to them relatively early. In other words, rather than deny them, or run from them, Bob directly faced his own health problems, including his asthma. About a year after the eventful cocktail party, Bob had this to say:

ॐ "My weight and blood pressure were easy to ignore, or 'deny,' as my wife would say. My pressure wasn't all that high, and neither was the weight; just high enough to bother me, I guess. What I've learned from this is that when I get bothered by something I try to ignore it, pretend it's not really a problem. That makes me feel less worried in the short run but can be a problem in the long run. When I started having trouble breathing, I just had to face it. It may have taken me a while, but I did face it.

"What happened was my doctor put me on some inhaled medicine for the asthma right away, and he gave me six months to get my weight down to see if that helped my blood pressure. If I didn't get my weight down, or if I did but the pressure was still too high, I'd have to go on medicine for that too. Well, I guess I took the whole thing as a challenge. I started by getting on a diet recommended by the American Diabetes Foundation. I don't have diabetes, thank goodness, but their diet appealed to me because it was pretty easy to follow, no nutrition mumbo jumbo. More like accounting, really. And I began exercising more than just my right wrist to change the channel on the TV. Nothing big, just two or three times a week in the gym, walking the treadmill, that sort of thing. Actually, don't tell Laurie, but I'm sort of addicted to that walking, and now I'm walking at the gym or outside almost five days a week.

"Anyway, within five months I had lost ten pounds, and for one reason or another my blood pressure was down into the almost normal range. So, no medicine needed there. And the best thing of all, I've been able to lower the asthma medicine too; my doctor says it's because it is easier for me to breathe with less weight on me. I guess that makes sense. Whatever the connection, my health résumé reads a little differently now. More strengths and fewer problems. I know I have to keep it up, but now I face my health every day rather than avoid it. One way or another I guess I have my asthma to thank for that."

Actually, we believe Bob has himself to thank for that!

Margaret's shift to a more adaptive mode of coping with her asthma also began with a revelation. It came not from her subconscious, as with Bob, but from someone she cared about very much.

  Margaret was a good, caring mother, and she prided herself on listening to her children. While getting ready to visit the pediatric allergist, her six-year-old refused to get dressed. "I'm not going," she angrily insisted. When Margaret asked why she was so mad and said it was only a doctor's appointment, it wouldn't hurt, and so forth, her daughter answered, "You're the one who's sick, not me." This hit Margaret like a ton of bricks, almost took her breath away, and she knew in that instant her daughter was right. It was she who needed help; the girls' doctor had as much as said so. Two phone calls later, she had canceled the allergist and made an appointment to see her own doctor instead. "Out of the mouths of babes," she thought.

It was not easy for Margaret to face her asthma. She didn't like the idea of having something wrong with her that would need regular attention, and she absolutely hated the idea that she might be limited to any degree in how she could care for or play with the girls. She made her concerns known to her doctor, and within a few months she had begun to face her asthma in a much more adaptive way. In her words:

  "Well, as you know, I learned from my own daughter that I wasn't paying enough attention to my asthma. Not the first thing I've learned from them, and not the last either. Really, now that I'm under way with a plan of treatment it's not as bad as I feared. My doctor says it will be several more months before we have the treatment plan down pat, and even then things will change depending on how I do, but for now at least I'm hanging in there. Yes, I take pills and use an inhaler every day, and sometimes I take extra treatments before I have to do something strenuous, but I can live with that, especially if that's what I need to do to be there for my family.

"I may have learned something from my daughter, but both girls still have a lot to learn from me. And one thing I want to teach them is how to take care of themselves socially, emotionally, and physically. What kind of a model was I setting by taking them to the doctor when I was ill? That's not what I want to model for them; I want to show them how to take care of themselves the best they can and not to let things get you down—get on with life, in other words. And I feel that's an important lesson I can give them by having them see how I take care of my asthma. Take care of yourself and get on with things—that's what I say."

What lessons can you take from Bob and Margaret? Consider at least these three:

1. *No matter how frightening the prospect of having asthma is, you have the courage to face the truth and the strength to change as necessary.* If you haven't yet figured out your own psychological defenses, when you get a nagging feeling like Bob did or a whack over the head like Margaret did, try to accept the revelation. Remind yourself that feeling fear does not mean you lack courage.

2. *Listen to those who know you well.* Try to keep an open mind, even if family and friends are telling you something you'd rather not hear. And don't forget to use them as sounding boards when your defenses are beginning to break down but have not yet crumbled: ask for the opinion of one you trust.

3. *Turn your defenses to a positive, adaptive purpose.* When Margaret began facing her asthma, she did not just give up her initial defensive response completely. Rather, she used it as a way to keep her motivated toward her own health care. She used her compliance with a program of regular medication and her occasional pretreatment before physically challenging events, like taking the girls swimming, as an opportunity to model good health care habits for the girls to follow. Margaret kept part of her caring defense in place, but it was no longer too much of a good thing. Now, her focus on the girls is part of a healthy, productive adaptation to her asthma.

DOWN THE ROAD TOWARD LIVING WELL WITH ASTHMA

Margaret's story illustrates mainly one dimension of adaptation: accepting asthma as part of your life so that you can deal with the changes it imposes. As we have emphasized, however, we want much more than that for you. By practicing ongoing self-awareness, using the techniques presented so far, and taking our practical tips for managing all the important areas of your life in the following chapters, you can live very well with asthma. In fact, hundreds of patients we've known have traveled this road and emerged with even richer lives than when they began.

No one is immune to the psychological impacts of stressful life events. No one is invulnerable. Whether the stress is medical (e.g., a recent diagnosis of asthma), financial, familial, or anything else, stress taxes our ability to function effectively. Following a significant life stressor, a temporary decline in our level of general functioning is almost inevitable. Furthermore, almost anything can be a stressor; what's easy for you may be difficult for me and vice versa. One person may cope relatively well with a changed financial status but fall apart at the idea of needing to see a doctor. For others, seeing their physician may be relatively stress free, but the thought of spending less money may be terrifying.

The most important thing to remember is that just as virtually anything may be experienced by an individual as a significant stressor, *any significant stressor also has the potential for an increased sense of personal efficacy and competence.* Bob's story is a good illustration of this process. When Bob stuck his head in the sand, his stubborn denial limited his ability to adapt effectively to the new life stressor of asthma. The fact that he did little to help himself or his situation certainly did not enhance his personal efficacy and competence.

Fortunately, that is not where Bob ended up. Bob did not just survive the crisis; he actually flourished. More than simply endure the diagnosis of asthma and all that it would entail, he went beyond it and made use of the stressor to improve his overall level of physical and psychological health. The steps he took were simple to identify, but they did take some hard work and perseverance to accomplish.

Bob, Margaret, and Troy each illustrate aspects of this healthy model of adaptation, one in which you can go beyond the diagnosis of asthma into an even healthier, more personally effective and competent way of life than before your asthma was diagnosed. First, know your defenses; they can be your ally but also your enemy. Second, capitalize on your strengths. If you are a caring person, care about yourself as Margaret did. If you are an information hound like Troy, become an expert on yourself and your asthma. Don't try to invent a new personality to cope with your asthma; rather, find the strengths in your present way of living and apply those to your new challenge. Third, rely on others. Bob relied on his wife for information about how he had coped in the past. Margaret relied on her daughters to hold up a mirror to what she was doing and why. Last, be active on your own behalf. This is a common thread in all of the examples in this chapter, and it is central to all people who flourish in the face of stress.

Good luck!

❧ PART III

FAMILY ADAPTATION TO ASTHMA

ᴈ Chapter 6

The Flexible Family

It is not just individuals who have an emotional response to asthma; families respond as well. Asthma can affect virtually every aspect of the family, from social and recreational life to vocational and financial stability, and even intimate relationships between spouses and between parents and their children. Your family can be your biggest source of support or your most dangerous minefield—frequently both. One person with asthma will affect all the other individual family members as well as the family unit itself. And conversely, how the nonasthmatic family members react will strongly affect the emotional adjustment of the asthmatic member. *When someone has asthma, the whole family can have trouble breathing.*

Jim is a forty-seven-year-old insurance salesman recently diagnosed with asthma. He is married and has two teenage sons. Jim's wife, Beth, talks about the impact of asthma on Jim and their family:

ᴈ "At first Jim's asthma didn't really affect him much. Or us. But as it worsened, the asthma prevented him from doing a lot of things around the house, even little things like taking out the trash. And it wasn't just hard on him; it affected all of us. For a while he kind of sulked, but I think he felt so unproductive he had to find something constructive to do. Since I had to do most of the heavy work, he started to help with the cooking and other lighter chores.

At first he didn't care for it much, but then one morning our son asked Jim to show him how to cook a Western omelet, and Jim couldn't have been more pleased. It was then I sensed the family was making some progress in coping with Jim's asthma."

Jim's discovery that he had asthma set into motion an alarming and unsettling but nevertheless somewhat predictable pattern of family events. Familiarity with that pattern can help you anticipate typical family problems and make adjustment to asthma more manageable. The goal of this chapter is to teach you to recognize such difficulties and to give you some suggestions for coping effectively.

All families are different, and each type of family environment presents a unique set of obstacles and offers unique opportunities for healthy adaptation. Where is your family in the complex process of adjustment? What kind of family do you have? What potential pitfalls can you foresee? What strengths can you all draw on? In the following pages we'll address these important questions.

DIAGNOSIS, RESPONSE, ADAPTATION

Just as it results in a complicated individual response, the diagnosis of asthma results in a complex family response, followed by a new level of adaptation. In fact, all major family events— marriage, the birth of a child, retirement—follow this pattern. The family unit responds, and a new level of adaptation results. If we can help you respond positively to the diagnosis of asthma, your family's adaptation will be a healthy one.

Diagnosis

&ev; Jim first noticed some shortness of breath when he was gardening or working around the house. Initially, he attributed the shortness of breath to being "out of shape." At forty-seven, Jim was fifteen pounds overweight and did little regular exercise. On the other hand, he did not smoke, he was generally healthy, with no history of breathing problems, and he did not suspect anything was seriously wrong. When his occasional shortness of breath turned into frequent wheezing, Beth suggested he see the family doctor. It was then that the diagnosis was made. However, it was not just Jim who received the diagnosis of asthma; his family received the news as well. At first, Jim and his family were relieved to hear it was "only asthma" (see the myths debunked in Chapter 1), but over the next few weeks they became increasingly concerned.

In this diagnostic phase of adjustment, your family is just as susceptible to myths, just as subject to uncertainty about asthma as you are. In Jim's family there was confusion about some medical terminology. Did Jim have asthma or exercise-induced bronchospasm (a type of asthma in which noticeable symptoms typically appear during exercise)? What exactly was asthma? Was it a serious illness? Few families know what asthma means for everyday life, what its causes are, how it is treated, and when it will go away when it enters their lives. Their understandable ignorance leaves them ripe for misconceptions, myths, and just plain bad information.

Many families turn first to doctors to inform them, but they often find they must look further to get all their questions answered. Finding an asthma doctor is not easy. Some health plans require an initial consultation with a family medicine physician before allowing you to see an allergist or a pulmonologist. And even then, just when you have the most questions, you may feel the most uneasy about asking for answers because you don't know the doctor very well. Nonetheless, good information is paramount, so be sure to find a physician who will provide the answers your family needs. Also, a variety of good books are available on the medical aspects of asthma (see the Appendix). Don't succumb to myths, and don't rely solely on your doctor for information. Educate yourself as well.

There is nothing easy about the diagnostic phase of asthma, for you or your family. Begin to talk as a family about the questions you have and how you can get them answered. Communication within the family is the key to adapting well to asthma. Begin that communication now.

Response

For your family, as for you, uncertainty is likely to result in fear, but there are as many other family responses to the diagnosis of asthma as there are individual responses. Emotionally, your family may feel frustrated, angry, sad, and guilty, as well as afraid. The one thing you may be certain of is that your family *will* respond and that response will likely be somewhat difficult at first. Pay attention to exactly how your family responds; it may be a clue to finding the place where things are going wrong when they do.

Initially, Jim responded to his fear about the diagnosis of asthma by denying that anything significant was wrong. His family followed suit. Some minor changes in lifestyle were made—for example, eating in the nonsmoking areas of restaurants—but for Jim, Beth, and their two sons it was still pretty much business as usual. As Jim's asthma worsened, though, so did his response and his family's. When his shortness of breath was too noticeable to deny, he sulked and did nothing useful to try to regain a sense of control over his health. As we discussed in Chapter 3, this left him feeling worthless and depressed, and the family too went through a period when the mood was quite gray. As family roles shifted, however, so did the mood of the family—for the better.

Because Jim couldn't take out the trash or mow the lawn, he began to cook. Now he felt more productive, and the family again saw him as a major contributor. Jim's son was used to looking up to his father, and when Jim stopped denying the asthma, ended his temporary strike, and started work again, Jim's son responded too. "I didn't know you could cook, Dad. Those Western omelets look great. Could you show me how to make one?"

Adaptation

Before asthma, Jim's family had relied on fairly traditional gender roles to divide up the work of the family. Jim was the wage earner and did the heavy work around the house. Beth was chief cook and bottle washer, and their sons modeled most of their activities on their father. The shift in family roles—Jim doing most of the cooking and Beth and the boys doing more of the heavy work—was an adaptation that seemed to work well for all of them. In a way it was especially useful for the boys, who now saw their parents in less traditional but broader ways. Shifting roles gave everybody new responsibilities that they were perfectly able to perform. Also, it gave the boys a wider range of attributes to admire and emulate in their father.

Change is usually difficult, and family changes are some of the most difficult to achieve. But you and your family can adapt to asthma. You can get through the difficult times. And sometimes, with effort, help, some luck, and a lot of humor, you and your family can not just survive but flourish. Adaptation means making positive changes so that the family is operating even better than before the diagnosis of asthma. Both individuals and the family can actually become stronger. So don't settle for just getting by. Your family has too much to gain. Later in this chapter we'll give you some ways to approach problems that do crop up in your family's adjustment, but first take the following success stories as inspiring examples of what you stand to gain by adapting as a family.

&ഝ Pete, a fifty-one-year-old accountant, and Cindy, his forty-four-year-old wife, both smoked cigarettes—three packs a day between them. Like every other smoker, they had been advised to quit, had tried to quit, but neither had ever been successful. Over the years, it was always Cindy who tried to get them to stop. She had enrolled them in antismoking classes, bought gum, the patch, and tried hypnosis. Pete would grudgingly go along with these efforts but, inevitably, when Cindy stopped smoking for a period Pete would continue, and after some time she would give in to the constant temptation of his smoking in front of her and start again. They had danced these steps several times over.

When Cindy was diagnosed with asthma, her doctor insisted that the most important aspect of her treatment would be to give up cigarettes. Cindy just didn't feel she had it in her to stop; after all, they had tried so many times in the past.

Pete was scared by Cindy's asthma. While he had been mildly concerned by all the health warnings about smoking, he had never been frightened enough to stop. This felt different. Pete was more worried about Cindy's health than he had ever been about his own. He was so scared he committed himself to getting her to stop smoking. Now their roles had changed, and so did the outcome. At Pete's suggestion they enrolled again in a support group, bought some nicotine gum, and also at Pete's urging, they quit cold turkey. Now that Pete was taking the lead Cindy was able to quit, and her asthma did improve almost immediately. The simple shift to Pete's being the initiator helped improve the health of both, and as a couple they were now functioning at a higher level than before the diagnosis of asthma.

In families adaptation often does mean role reversal, and sometimes that's what causes the family to flourish.

ਏ Typical of many couples with young children, Marianne and John Clarkson had watched their sexual activity diminish until they were making love only about once a month. Generally, they didn't have sex at all unless John initiated it, and they rarely discussed their sex life directly.

When John was diagnosed with asthma, his doctor suggested that changes in his types of physical exertion might be necessary, including sexual activity. Because their doctor brought up the topic, John and Marianne found themselves a little more able to discuss their sexual relationship openly. When John admitted he was afraid his asthma would mean their sexual encounters would be even less frequent, Marianne decided to make a change in her role, namely, she decided to become more of the initiator of sex, and they both tried some of the suggestions for experimenting with different positions outlined in Chapter 7. Within three months of his diagnosis of asthma, John and Marianne were making love weekly, not monthly, and overall the whole family seemed happier.

ਏ The Wilkensons spent much of their free time supporting fifteen-year-old Benny in his various sports. He enjoyed playing football, basketball, and baseball for his school even though he was not a starter for any of the teams. When his asthma worsened to the point that competing became more difficult, the only person who didn't seem thrown was Benny. His parents jovially assured him they'd "work it out with the doctor" and have Benny "back on the field in no time," but Benny caught their worried, sympathetic glances when they thought he wasn't looking. Finally, when he couldn't stand any more, Benny confronted them: "Look, Mom and Dad, if you care so much about sports, why don't *you* play? I don't think I can handle it right now." Benny's parents were stunned. They assured him they had only been worried about his feelings and couldn't care less about sports—it was Benny they cared about. They all agreed that Benny should try some other activities for a year, until Benny had had time to get his asthma under control.

A year later, nobody could argue that Benny's role as Captain Vere in the play *Billy Budd* was a huge success. He was finally first string. Also, his family had found other events to occupy their free time, although they never missed one of his shows.

Role shifting, communication, flexibility, fairness—the preceding families exhibited many qualities essential to family adaptation. Note, however, that they all had to make rather dramatic changes because of the severity of the asthma. If your asthma is less severe, the necessary family changes will also be less dramatic.

In either case, *always make changes gradually and only as needed.* Rather than changing roles entirely, slight shifts in lifestyle may be all that is necessary. Start with small changes and build to larger ones only as it becomes clear that they are truly needed. For example, before giving the household chores entirely to Beth, Jim could try modifying the chores, finding ways to make them easier before giving them up altogether. Maybe he could still take out the trash, for example, if the can had wheels.

A good rule of thumb is to find the places where your family gets stuck and do some creative problem solving to get the family moving again. You'll be well prepared to do that on demand if you understand what kind of family you live in.

A FAMILY ANALYSIS: PREPARING FOR CHANGE

What are your family's typical ways of coping with stress, of managing change, of promoting physical and emotional health? Although all families go through the pattern of diagnosis, response, and adaptation, each family passes through those stages in its own special way. One family might appear quite stoic:

→ "Stressed by my asthma? We are the Smithbacks," said a fifty-year-old woman to her physician. "We are rarely stressed, and when we are we don't take it sitting down. We fight back. Smithbacks don't spend much time worrying about themselves. We can all take care of ourselves."

Another family may take a much less aggressive stance toward asthma. In the Frank family, the tone was very different:

→ "Everyone seemed to get closer when Mom's asthma got worse. We'd do everything around the house and take care of her too. Unfortunately, if she got depressed or angry we all seemed to get depressed and angry too."

How the Smithbacks and Franks cope with a family member's asthma depends not just on which phase of asthma they are in but also on the type of family they are in general. Learn to recognize your type of family.

Family Types

The "perfect family" for an asthmatic to live in has the following characteristics. Family members are emotionally close, communicate well, are understanding, respectful, and supportive of each other. Members are close, but they are not too close. People are able to maintain their own privacy, and there is respect for individual differences and personal autonomy. The individual members of the family are flexible, adaptable, and willing to try new roles when needed. And the family unit as a whole is flexible, adaptable, and willing to shift roles and responsibilities without throwing the whole family into chaos.

Sounds great, doesn't it? That's because the perfect family for an asthmatic to live in is the perfect family for anyone to live in. Unfortunately, *perfect families do not exist!* Every family is unique, with its own strengths and weaknesses. Every family goes through times when communication between members is especially good and other times when it's hard to feel understood even about very simple things. Support for autonomy, flexibility, and willingness to try changes comes and goes.

Fortunately, *you do not need a perfect family to adapt to asthma.* What you do need is a family that is willing to look at itself and determine if some of the ways the family operates are not good for you. Are family members so close that they worry too much about you? Is the family so busy that you don't feel listened to or supported? Once you have an understanding of what is not working in your family, you can try some of our suggestions for making healthy, adaptive changes that will benefit not just you but also the rest of your family.

Here are two common types of families that have gone too far in the direction of closeness or individuality. Families that go too far in any one direction can become rigid and difficult to change.

Too Close-Knit

Some families try to help each other too much. Family members may be so close that they don't have enough privacy, and individuals may feel they are being told how they should feel about their asthma. Family members feel so close that they can smother each other with affection and care. At times that may feel good, but not to most asthmatics, most of the time. *People with asthma need to breathe.*

Joel is a thirty-five-year-old computer operator whose family worries about his asthma a great deal, perhaps too much. As Joel says:

> "Sure, my wife takes care of me—does she ever! Whenever I'm ready to do something around the house, mow the lawn, for instance, she jumps all over me. 'How do you feel? Are you sure you feel up to it? Did you use your inhaler? Maybe you should wait until the wind dies down. Don't overdo it.' It makes me so mad I'm usually short of breath before I get out the door."

Rebecca finds herself in a similar situation:

    ⁕ "I'm fifty years old. I've raised a family, managed a household, taught school for fifteen years, and I'm very active in the community. I'm respected socially and professionally as a competent, intelligent woman. But around my family I sometimes feel like a helpless, stupid child. They check whether I've taken treatments, like I have no memory of my own. They smother me with attention, like I'm a complete invalid. The first thing I hear in the morning isn't 'Good morning.' It's 'How do you feel?' I think I would feel better if they would just get off my back."

Some close-knit families tend to be overprotective as well. With all their good intentions, families or individuals who are overprotective may undermine your sense of personal competency by implying that you cannot properly care for yourself. Being overprotected may feel like an attack on your own sense of control over your illness, and you may feel angered at the implication that you need so much help. Or you may actually come to feel you *cannot* care adequately for yourself. Neither anger and resentment nor passive acceptance of unneeded help is a healthy stance for a person with asthma. As a result, individual creativity, flexibility, and problem solving may diminish—not only within the asthmatic but also in the whole family. "If they do so much for me, it must mean they think I can't do it myself" becomes a tacit understanding of everyone when overprotectiveness toward any one member is established as the norm.

If some people in your family feel they have to take care of your illness for you, don't let them. Set limits on what they can and cannot do for you. Show them you can care for yourself. Be careful, however, not just to talk a good game. If you miss treatments, don't eat properly, forget to exercise, or push yourself too hard, you are wearing a big placard that says, "Regardless of what I might say I want, please take care of me. I won't do it for myself."

Again, smothering often begins with the best intentions. Many families draw together in times of crisis, and that's how your asthma might be perceived. The fact that asthma can make close families even closer has its advantages. If asthma places limitations on your social life, it can be a comfort to have family members with whom to spend time. And if that time together is spent in pursuit of true adaptation and mutual support, it's time well spent. But if the topic of asthma begins to play too big a role in family discussions, you run the risk of turning into "The Asthma Family." Continue to be the Smiths, the Martinellis, or the Cliens—a family with one member who has asthma.

Don't let asthma smother your family; everyone in the family needs room to breathe.

Too Independent

In these families, in contrast, the members are very separate and relatively unconnected. Quite the opposite of smothering families, individuals in these families may feel alone, lacking any support from each other.

People in families that are too independent may tend to ignore the asthma altogether, expecting the asthmatic to lead the same lifestyle as everyone else. The most important thing to remember about people who ignore your asthma is that they downplay the illness because of how it makes *them* feel. When you hurt, they hurt, and so by ignoring your pain they can feel better themselves. Remember, your family is probably ignoring your asthma because of the pain of caring, not because they "just don't care."

The Becks are typical of overly independent families. June Beck talks about how hard it is to face her husband's asthma:

> "I know Tom feels I don't pay enough attention to his breathing problems, asthma, reactive airways, whatever they call it. The psychologist asked me why I wasn't sure what my husband's diagnosis was. The truth is I'd rather not know. I'd rather not think about it at all. I guess that's my way of not letting it get to me. The kids take their lead from me. Maybe we're kidding ourselves, but it's hard to think about someone you love not being able to breathe."

Both Tom and June work hard, the kids are busy at school, and all of the family members tend to go their own way. Their independence from each other means they may not be used to asking for or giving direct help and support. They don't love each other any less; it is just the way their family operates best.

Having a diagnosis of your family type should make it easier to ask for what you need, to be flexible enough to solicit change in your family and make changes of your own. If you're a member of a family that is overly independent, for example, alter your own outlook to recognize that asking for help and support you need is a sign of strength, not weakness.

Flexibility: Managing Change

Adaptation to asthma depends on the family's willingness to consider changing. Yet like most stresses on family life, asthma makes families more rigid in the way they solve problems. That means that under a stress like asthma, your family may hold fiercely to its modus operandi *even if it is obviously not working well.*

If your usual way of handling family stress isn't working for asthma, try some new ways. If the old ways of looking after each other are making it harder for you to breathe, be flexible and try something new. If your family feels smothering, let them know, take good care of yourself, and ask for more breathing room. If your family feels too detached, don't just wish for more support; communicate your needs and ask for the specific kind of help or support you want. Later in this chapter we'll suggest ways to ease the problems that asthma causes in families, but for now, remember: Stay flexible—it's easier to breathe that way!

Trying On Another Point of View

The first place to practice flexible thinking is in how you see whatever is going wrong. Regardless of what type of family you have, the first step in adapting to asthma in the family is always the same: Look at the situation from the other person's point of view. If someone is smothering you, see it as a sign of his or her wish to help. If family members ignore your asthma, see if their attitude is caused by their pain at watching you have trouble breathing. Whatever the problem, family members usually think they are doing something to help the asthmatic and the whole family. If you can see each difficulty from the other family members' points of view, you will understand your family better, and problems will immediately seem easier to solve. Then, let them know you understand some of what they face and how *your* asthma gives *them* problems. That alone will go a long way toward getting the family on the right track again.

Changing Family Roles

For most families, asthma requires a shifting of roles and responsibilities, from household chores to sexual positions. Role changes in the family always lead to a temporary sense of disorganization, but ironically, this time of family turmoil can also be an important time of positive change. The family's level of rigidity is temporarily low, and flexibility (disguised as chaos!) is high. So don't wait for things to settle down before beginning the work of adapting to new roles. Start while things are at their most unsettled. Benetta, a thirty-seven-year-old wife and mother of three small children, talks about the mistake of waiting too long:

> ঌ "When my husband's asthma started getting worse, everything changed. He was forced to give up his weekend job because the work was too strenuous. I suggested maybe it was my turn to take a second job—tutoring, even weekend typing—but he said, 'No, let's wait until things settle down.' Well, we waited, and I passed up some jobs in the process. The only thing that's settled now is that his asthma is worse, and we are poorer."

A family that successfully adapts to asthma may end up functioning even better than before, but the process can be hard, and it takes time. Shifting roles often leaves people with temporary feelings of uselessness, sadness, and anger. Pay attention to how all family members are feeling when role shifts are necessary. And again, make the shifts gradually and keep the balance. If there are things you cannot do, find things you can do (even if you don't especially like doing them). In other words, if asthma means you must give up some things, add some new things to your life. Remember Jim and the Western omelet.

A word about free time: no one has enough, and as roles shift in your family free time may now be taken up with additional chores and responsibilities. Don't let this happen. Yes, it is important to take on new roles, but it is equally important to have some free time for yourself and for the family as a whole. You need time to do what you want, and time for the family to be together and do what it wants. The only way to get *any* free time is to make it an individual and a family priority.

COMMUNICATION: SUSTAINING FAMILY RELATIONSHIPS

While you're busy shifting roles and points of view to keep the family functioning smoothly, don't forget about those individual relationships that make up the family. No matter how flexible you are, your whole family will suffer if your marriage is shaken by asthma or if problems fester between you and your children of any age. Keep the lines of communication open and you can spot problems before they become big trouble.

Your Marriage

If you have asthma, it will be obvious to all of your loved ones that you're suffering. But it is important to remember that your spouse suffers also, and too often in silence. Spouses of asthmatics may feel frustrated, angry, depressed, let down and alone. In short, your spouse is susceptible to the same range of painful feelings as you are but may feel less able to express those feelings directly out of fear of making you feel worse. Usually, that won't happen. The truth is, you probably already feel guilty about the changes in family and marital life caused by your illness.

Directly discussing your mate's negative feelings can help create a sense of openness and even relief from some of that burden of guilt. Diana, for example, worries about how her husband, Ted, really feels about her asthma:

> ⁚ "I know that my asthma is a problem for Ted. The house isn't kept as nicely as he'd like. I don't feel up to doing as much; in the bedroom I'm not as interested. He's so understanding it makes me feel more guilty. Sometimes I wish he'd just blow up at me and let me know exactly how he feels. In a funny way I think I'd feel better."

Marriage is a balance, and guilt can tip the balance unnecessarily. Both partners dread being a burden. If you are the healthy spouse of an asthmatic, find some ways to help ease your mate's sense of being a burden. The best way to do this is not by helping him or her more but by finding ways to let your spouse help you. If your mate can help you, he or she may be better able to accept your help in return. Thus, the balance is restored.

Dealing with the Gender Gap

Sounds pretty simple, doesn't it? Of course, it may not be, because men and women tend to deal with asthma differently. If you are already a thoroughly "liberated" male—comfortable with feelings, ready to ask for help, and not afraid to be soft and sensitive—ignore this next section. Likewise, if you are a woman who feels no discomfort at being assertive, if you're comfortable being strong and independent, you don't need to read this section. Frankly, though, even in this enlightened age most of us still slip occasionally into stereotypical male or female roles. So it will probably be helpful to read on. Traditionally, men and women really do tend to deal with asthma differently, and these differences are important to recognize and cope with for your sake as well as the sake of your spouse and family.

Many men have a difficult time coping with the increased emotionality that often accompanies asthma. Listen to Sam, a forty-year-old cook:

ச் "The thing I hate about asthma is how I can't control my feelings. I get mad one minute, sad the next, and mostly I just never know *how* I'm going to feel. Before I had asthma I was pretty good at putting my feelings aside and just doing what had to be done; now I seem to have lost control of them completely. It's not the breathing that bothers me; it's the crying."

Men are frequently uncomfortable with strong feelings, but asthma creates strong feelings in almost everyone. As discussed in Chapter 3, if you are a man with asthma and your feelings are getting the better of you, there are steps you can take. Name the feelings, face those feelings directly, eliminate irrational thoughts, challenge yourself to feel your emotions, and then move on.

For a woman the difficulty may not be coping with strong feelings but assertively asking for needed help. Jane is a housewife about the same age as Bob. She is uneasy asking her husband and family for what she needs:

ச் "My friends tell me I should ask for more help from my husband and kids so I won't have to do it all myself. I wouldn't mind if they helped around the house more, of course. I just hate having to ask them. I feel so guilty, like I'm not carrying my weight anymore. My daughter says I need to be more assertive, but that's not how I was raised, and that's not who I am."

Different demands and stresses may occur depending on whether it is the husband or wife who has asthma. When the husband has asthma, for example, it may be very important to strengthen the wife's other roles to help her balance the increased time she spends caring for her husband. Because her husband has asthma, the wife will tend to spend more time providing nurturance, care, and support than she might if her husband had no breathing problems. However, too much care*giving* and not enough care*taking* may lead the wife to feel angry and resentful toward her asthmatic husband. Furthermore, if she feels angry at her sick husband, she may end up feeling guilty as well.

To prevent unhelpful feelings of anger, resentment, and guilt from building, the wife of an asthma patient must do more for herself as well as doing more for her asthmatic husband. If you work out of the home, emphasize your work; don't neglect it. Enhance your work by expanding your areas of competence and enjoyment. Take a seminar designed to make you a better, more valued employee. Or take a class just to get you out of the house doing something that interests you and that you enjoy. Spend more time with your friends, not less. In other words, if you are the wife of an asthma patient, don't just take of your husband; *take care of yourself!*

Kathleen is a thirty-two-year-old administrative assistant whose husband has asthma. She found herself in the familiar trap of spending too much time caring for those around her. Then Kathleen did something about it:

ဆ "As my husband's asthma got worse, I found myself practically shut off from the outside world. At work, I spent the day taking care of my boss. Then I'd come home and spend half the night taking care of my husband. It wasn't that my husband wasn't appreciative; it just seemed that the more I supported him and his asthma, the madder I got. Pretty soon I was snapping at him, snapping at my coworkers, and not enjoying much of anything. It was funny; he was the one with the breathing problem, but I was the one having trouble coping.

"My sister suggested I take a cooking class I'd been interested in. At first, I resisted; where would I find the time? Eventually I gave in, and it really helped—and not just with my cooking. I found that one night out a week doing something just for me made the rest of the week go much better."

Patterns of caregiving in the family may also be problematic when the wife has asthma and the husband does not. Men sometimes have a tendency to push, prod, or goad their spouses into feeling better. Men may believe the myth that if only the asthma patient tried harder she would breathe better. If your wife has asthma, she may even act like this strategy is working (to get you off her back), but it probably does not help much in the long run. Most people feel worse after being prodded, not better. A husband who wants to help his asthmatic wife needs simply to ask his wife how best to help. Don't *tell* your wife to breathe better; *help* her breathe better.

Men may tend to put family concerns second, whereas women might place them first. If your asthma demands that your husband help and support you more than he is accustomed to, don't imagine that he will change simply because you have asthma. It's up to you to figure out what you need from your husband. Once you know what you need, educate your spouse about those needs—emotional, physical, sexual, social. Then, since you're asking him for something additional, find something you can do for him in return. You may think you do enough already, but to keep the balance find something new.

Educating your spouse need not be difficult or burdensome. It may be best to "strike while the iron is cold"; in other words, talk about your needs when things are going well between the two of you rather than during a fight or when feelings are tense. When we ask others for help, they are more likely to be receptive if they feel appreciated for what efforts they have made, not attacked for their shortcomings. Talk to your spouse while out on a date, during a leisurely meal, or during some quiet time the two of you are spending together. Never try to educate your spouse when the television is on, when the children are around, or when you don't have each other's undivided attention. Finally, make your needs easy to understand, and communicate them clearly and briefly. In fact, having several brief conversations, ten minutes or so long, when the two of you are together, uninterrupted, and getting along, is a good recipe for marital communication about almost any important topic, including your needs stemming from your asthma.

Your Children

Just as you worry about the effects of your illness on your mate, you will have concerns about the possible negative impact on your children. How will you come up with the time, energy, attention, money, and understanding that children need when asthma seems to be such a drain on those quantities? How will having a sick parent emotionally affect your child's development? Will your children think less of you for being physically limited? Will they think you're inadequate?

Yes, your children will respond, even quite strongly, to your asthma. But how they respond depends in large part on how *you* respond to your asthma. In other words, it's not your asthma that the children respond to but, rather, how you manage your asthma. Communicating to your children that you have asthma may be relatively easy. If they are old enough to understand, bring them in on the diagnostic phase. What lasts and is ultimately of the most importance, however, is communicating to your children a model of realistic self-care. Show them (instead of just telling them) how to face, manage, and even flourish in the face of life's unwanted visitors. Twelve-year-old Sharon spoke about her mother with asthma:

> ❧ "I know Mom feels like she's letting me down sometimes, like not helping with cheerleading or how she gets attacks sometimes at my field hockey games. But I don't really feel that way. I've told her that stuff isn't as important to me as she thinks. To tell you the truth, the only time I really feel let down by her is when she gets sick because she does too much and doesn't have the sense to slow down."

Young Children

Whether your children are five, fifteen, or fifty-five, it can be difficult on them to see you suffer from asthma. It is helpful to consider the age of your children when deciding how to help them cope with your asthma. For example, young children may have trouble understanding your asthma and may be secretly fearful that you may die from it. Also, young children tend to see themselves as the center of the universe, responsible for all that happens, good or bad. So they may believe that somehow they caused your illness, by being "bad" or making you work so hard picking up after them. Always try to explain to your children that asthma is serious but can be managed. Asthma is not caused by them, but you do need their help in dealing with it. They may understand more than you think.

Finally, if reassuring and explaining do not help, *show them* that you can manage your asthma. Showing them will go a long way toward reassuring them that you're not going to die or be angry with them because of your asthma.

Don't make the mistake of confusing love with activity. You may not be able to do as much with your children physically, but that doesn't mean that you love them any less, and they will understand that. How much strenuous activity you do together is no more a gauge of how much you love them than is how many things you can buy them. It is the quality of the time together that counts, not the quantity. Your asthma may present a wonderful opportunity to teach this lesson too easily forgotten by most of us.

Once again, the formula for success is the same:

1. Acknowledge your asthma to yourself and then to your children.
2. Know what your needs are, and know your limitations.
3. Communicate those needs and limits to your children, and ask directly for their help in meeting them.
4. Don't do things with your children that don't fit for you; children don't need the guilt that goes with knowing that they pushed Mom or Dad too far. Spend the kind of quality time with your children that meets your needs, and you will likely find it meets many of theirs as well.

Parents with asthma may also be concerned that they will pass their asthma on to their children. Chapter 8 discusses the specific concerns of childhood asthma. Although you cannot "infect" someone with asthma, there is a strong genetic component. If one parent has asthma, the chances of a child having asthma are about twenty-five percent. If both parents have asthma, the chances go up to forty to sixty percent. Of course, there is little you can do about your children's genes at this point, so instead of worrying about things you cannot control, focus on those things you can. Keep a dust-free, smoke-free environment, and focus on your relationship with your children, not your guilt about having asthma. Your children may or may not have asthma now or in the future; that is beyond your control.

Your children are learning how to cope with asthma, and other problems of adult life, by watching you live with your asthma. Do you hide it from yourself and others or confront it directly and attempt to master it? Do you understand the physiology and psychology of your asthma and the effects it has on you and your family? Or do you remain ignorant, passive, and thereby force others to manage your asthma for you? These are the lessons your children are learning. Don't spend time worrying about your children's genetic inheritance; worry about the examples you set for them every day.

Adolescents

Adolescents with an asthmatic parent may need special care. Most teenagers want to have *less* to do with their parents and spend *less* time at home in general. Because of a parent's asthma, however, the adolescent may be asked to help more around the house and be more attuned to the parent's physical and emotional needs. As a result, the adolescent may become angry and resentful.

If your adolescent is having a hard time coping with your asthma and the demands it places on his or her life, start by acknowledging that you understand that you're asking the child to do things that he or she would prefer not to do. Second, if you require more, grant the teenager some additional privileges in return. Like the marital relationship, the parent–child relationship must maintain its balance. If you ask more, give more. Also, remember that you're dealing with a near adult. Don't lecture the teen about asthma; let your son or daughter read about it. Give him or her this book and one or two that focus on the medical aspects of the illness (see the Appendix). Finally, and most important, if you want teenagers to respond in a mature way, treat them as the adults they almost are. Adolescents may pretend not to care and seem concerned only about how your asthma affects their independence. Don't believe it; they just act as if they don't care as a way of building their own sense of who they are, separate from their parents.

Adult Children

Adult children may have a different kind of fear. Adult children may see your asthma as a sign of general decline in your health, signaling your old age and death. They really may be very concerned about your health and may need some straight talk with you about asthma, your health in general, and how you plan to care for yourself in your most senior years. Most adult children worry about their parents' health—there is nothing unusual about that. Make sure they understand how your asthma fits into your health picture, and show them how well it can be managed.

If your adult children become too concerned, they may act just like the overly close or overly independent families described earlier. Some adult children will become overprotective and even intrusive. Others may back off, not offering the help and support you need. In either case, the strategy for coping is the same: Identify what it is about their response that causes you problems, know your own needs, then openly communicate those needs for more space, more help, or both.

Your asthma may also remind your adult children of their own health concerns. After all, they are getting older too. Problems with health become more of a concern as we get older, and your adult children are like anyone else; people prefer not to think about health problems and mortality in general. If your asthma reminds your children about their own health, they may tend to withdraw from you emotionally, spending less time with you and providing less support for your asthma. If you notice this pattern, help your children face their fears by showing how you face yours. Talk with your adult children about your own fears about asthma and illness in general, and invite them to do the same.

In general, *the best way to take care of your children is to take good care of yourself.*

EVOLUTION AND GROWTH: UNDERSTANDING THE FAMILY LIFE CYCLE

Complicating matters of adaptation somewhat is that family relationships are, of course, not static. For your family to adapt to asthma you must recognize where you are in the family life cycle—the usual course of events and demands faced by most families across time. One family life cycle might go like this: marriage, the birth and raising of children, career building, children leaving home and getting married themselves, parents eventually retiring, death of one generation, and birth of children into the next. Not all families face each of these events, and not always in this order, but most families go through a similar pattern.

All major events in the family life cycle are stressful, and all require the family to respond and adapt. If you're not convinced of this, ask yourself these questions: Was it stressful planning our wedding? Did we need to adapt to the new baby? What about raising a teenager—stressful? How about going to work every day, planning for retirement? All important events, even good ones, are stressful to the family. Asthma is no different; it is an important and troubling event in any family's life cycle. To adapt successfully to asthma you must recognize where in the family life cycle your asthma hits. For example, if the twenty-five-year-old mother of a new baby has asthma, the effects on the family are very different than for the family of a sixty-five-year-old man getting ready to retire. Where is your family in its life cycle? How does asthma affect family life at your place in the cycle?

Early Family Life

People in their twenties and thirties are usually in the beginning stages of adult family life. No longer a child in your own family of origin, you are now free to explore life's adult options and begin to build a family life of your own. Raising children and building a career are your priorities. If this is where you are in the family life cycle, asthma presents some particular challenges. As a young family you may have had little need to adapt to a chronic stress such as asthma. Now, asthma threatens to upset the kind of healthy, active family lifestyle you had always envisioned. But you have coped with other family stresses (children, jobs, home), and by bringing those flexible skills to bear your family can adapt to asthma as well.

It may anger and disappoint you and your family when someone's asthma intrudes into the raising of your children, the advancing of your careers, or in any way interferes with the active lifestyle you had envisioned. As a result, the asthmatic person in this stage of the family life cycle may feel especially burdensome to the family. Yes, asthma can be a burden at this stage, but that doesn't mean the family's lifestyle need be burdened or depressed. For every family event that asthma limits, there is more time for the family to spend together in some other quality way. Camping may be out, but walking is in. Roughhousing with the kids may be difficult, but more story time can be a pleasure for the whole family. Yes, some physical activities may be limited, but the quality time spent together can still be enjoyed. You must acknowledge your limitations and then focus on what you can still do together as a family.

How you respond and adapt to asthma may serve as a model for how you cope with life's future hurdles. Asthma can pull your family apart or bring you together. Limiting some activities does not mean reducing your commitment to each other. This first phase of the family life cycle sets the tone for all that follows; make that tone a positive one.

The Midlife Family

For families at midlife, when the adults are roughly forty to sixty-five, the challenge of asthma is quite different. Now that the pressure to "get going" with your family and careers has

eased, you have more time to take a look at your life, your values, and where you want to go from here. Children are moving out and beginning families of their own. You may find yourself asking uncomfortable questions: What have I accomplished so far? Is my family and work life rewarding? Where do we go from here?

At this stage you may struggle between wanting to stand pat and coast toward grandchildren and retirement and continuing to grow, individually and as a family. An asthmatic person may feel tempted to stand pat. It's hard work to grow and achieve when you're short of breath. You may want to say, "I've achieved, I've got a steady job, the kids are on their own. Why keep pushing?" Be careful; the family that gives in to asthma at this stage may cheat itself out of the best years of family life.

Now, more than ever, you must be active in family life and social life, at home and in the community. You may even be tempted to use your asthma as an excuse to plant roots in the easy chair. Well, if you're going to turn into a couch potato at age fifty-five, don't blame it on your asthma.

If you look back at your family's life with asthma and don't like what you see, *change it now*. If you have hidden your asthma from your family and now you regret it, *let them in*. If you haven't spent enough quality time with those you love, *spend that time now*. It's not too late to change—unless you keep putting it off. When you look back on your family's adaptation to asthma, you may recall this midlife stage the best; make it something to remember.

Late-Adult Family Life

Now, your children have children, you have retired, and you're supposed to be old and wise. You may still feel young and immature, but others look to you as someone who should know how to handle most of life's problems. What does it mean to have asthma at this stage? Like other physical problems you may be coping with, asthma may interfere with plans for the retirement you had hoped for. As at any phase of the family life cycle,

physical activities such as golf, for example, may be too difficult. You can, however, find other ways to spend your new leisure time with those you care about most. Having asthma at this stage of family life should not affect your intellectual, social, and community pursuits. Once again, if you're considering a retreat to the couch, don't blame it on your asthma.

You can view asthma as a sign of decline or another instance of your successful adaptation to life's challenges. Asthma itself means very little; how you manage your asthma is what counts. Age does not ensure knowledge or healthy adaptation. The family will still struggle and must use its resources to adapt, as at any other stage. You owe it to yourself to be as flexible as you can. Flexibility at this stage of family life may really be what "older and wiser" is all about.

CREATIVITY: FAMILY PROBLEM-SOLVING TECHNIQUES

Many of the difficulties that asthma has caused your family can be solved by simply recognizing that a problem exists, diagnosing the causes of that problem, viewing the problem from the other person's point of view, and then taking the commonsense steps that seem called for. The general advice we've given so far can go a long way toward circumventing problems at home. When something specific proves stubborn, however, you might try these tried-and-true techniques:

Six Steps to Problem Solving

Sometimes families feel so stuck that a more organized approach may be needed. Here are some suggestions for solving those particularly sticky family problems:

1. *Plan a family meeting.* When family conflicts come up, you may want to say, "That's one for the next family meeting." Don't always try to solve problems right when they come up;

tempers may be too hot and thinking too rigid. Meet for a set amount of time (thirty minutes should do) and work on only one problem at each meeting.

2. *Agree that the problem is a family problem.* For that thirty minutes, everyone must agree that the problem belongs to the whole family, and so everyone must work together to solve it. It is not Dad's problem coping with his asthma, or Mom's anger at having to do more work around the house, or Jimmy's refusal to take out the garbage. It is the Jones family's problem, and all of the Joneses must work on it together.

3. *State the problem clearly.* Be very specific. What behavior, attitude, or tone of voice is troubling? Everyone must state his or her own view of the family problem and how he or she feels about it.

4. *Now, state the problem from the other person's point of view.* This step is the heart of the matter and is sometimes referred to as "active listening." Everyone in the family now must state the specific family problem from all points of view. This will be both fun and enlightening.

5. *Be flexible.* Discuss the pros and cons of as many possible solutions to the family problem as everyone can think of. Then, compromise on one solution, and give it a set amount of time for a trial period. Finally . . .

6. *Check back.* Meet again as a family to discuss how the trial solution is working. Are parts of it working well but others not? Does it need to be scrapped altogether, or is it working well enough? Congratulate yourselves on a good job.

A Problem-Solving Example

Here is an example of the right way and the wrong way to use the six steps of family problem solving. The Abbots seemed to have a fight every Wednesday night, trash night. Mr. Abbot's severe asthma prevented him from doing such heavy jobs as collecting, bagging, and carrying the trash to the curb. As a result, every Wednesday night Mrs. Abbot did the trash, and every Wednesday night Mrs. Abbot got angry. The two Abbot children, ages five and seven, were just too young to handle the chore themselves. How should they proceed?

৵ 1. PLAN A FAMILY MEETING.

Right Way: After a couple of months of "Wednesday night at the fights," as seven-year-old John called it, the Abbots decided to have a family meeting the following Friday evening from 7:30 to 8:00 P.M.

Wrong Way: On the Wednesday before the family meeting another fight broke out. Mr. Abbot yelled, "I'm sick of all this fighting. We're a family. Let's sit down and work this out right now!" Wrong, Mr. Abbot; tempers are too hot, especially yours. Your family has picked a time to problem-solve; wait until then.

৵ 2. AGREE THAT THE PROBLEM IS A FAMILY PROBLEM.

Right Way: Everyone agreed that the problem of the trash was, for that thirty minutes, a family problem, and everyone would work on it together.

Wrong Way: Mrs. Abbot suggested that the kids could skip the meeting because they were too young to solve the problem since they couldn't do the trash themselves. No, Mrs. Abbot; this problem affects everyone and needs to be solved by everyone.

৵ 3. STATE THE PROBLEM CLEARLY.

Right Way: First, everyone stated the problem from his or her own point of view. Mr. Abbot said he felt useless at not being able to do the garbage. Mrs. Abbot said she was angry that such an unpleasant job always fell to her. Mary (age five) said the problem was that she felt scared when her parents fought.

Together, after hearing all the points of view, the Abbots decided that the problem was how to get the trash out every week without any angry, sad, hurt, or scared feelings.

Wrong Way: Mr. Abbot said, "I know; it's my asthma that is the problem here." No, Mr. Abbot; the problem is not your asthma. The problem is the trash and those angry, sad, hurt, or scared feelings.

⅏ 4. NOW, STATE THE PROBLEM FROM THE OTHER PERSON'S POINT OF VIEW.

Right Way: For example, seven-year-old John was able to say, "I get it. Dad feels like a couch potato when Mom does the trash. Mom feels like a slave when she has to do all the dirty work, and Mary gets scared when you two fight, because she thinks it means you'll get divorced or something." Nice work, John.

Wrong Way: Mrs. Abbot got off to a rocky start with this step when she said, "You kids just want to get out of work. Your father at least has an excuse." At this point Mr. Abbot, John, and even Mary had to help Mrs. Abbot see the problem from each of their points of view.

⅏ 5. BE FLEXIBLE.

Right Way: The Abbots came up with several possible solutions, everything from doing the garbage every other week to collecting the garbage every day, so it would be in small enough amounts for the kids to do it themselves, and even the idea of a "garbage party," when the Abbots would invite their neighbors over to help and serve juice and cookies (Mary's idea). They discussed the advantages and disadvantages of each possible solution, and here is what they decided.

Mr. Abbot would be in charge of the trash. He couldn't physically collect it, but it was his job to make sure it got done. He felt good about this. John and Mary were responsible for collecting their own garbage, as well as the small trash bin in each bathroom. This was more than they were used to, but if it stopped the fighting it seemed worthwhile. Mrs. Abbot was still in charge of collecting the larger trash cans, and she still took it all to the curb. However, every Wednesday night Mrs. Abbot was relieved of kitchen duty. Mr. Abbot would cook (or order pizza), and Mr. Abbot, John, and Mary would all clean the kitchen. Mrs. Abbot secretly thought she was getting the best deal of all and felt much less angry. The Abbots agreed to meet again in one month to see how things were working out.

Wrong Way: At first the family could think of only one or two possible solutions, and they were tempted to settle for "Take out the trash every other week." This plan would not have worked. It wasn't until Mary's trash-party idea loosened things up that the family got more flexible in their thinking.

✎ 6. *CHECK BACK.*

Right Way: In one month, the plan needed only minor revisions. Mrs. Abbot said that pizza every Wednesday night was too often, and they agreed on pizza only once a month. Aside from that the plan seemed good enough.

Wrong Way: After a couple of weeks, Mr. Abbot wanted to jump the gun. "This plan works great," he declared at dinner one evening. "Why even meet again?" "Oh, no," said Mary. "That's not fair. We have to meet again for the check-in." And so they did.

The Abbots found a healthy new way of working together, not just in regard to asthma but also as a family in general. So can you.

ꙩ Chapter 7

A Healthy Sex Life with Asthma

Because asthma can affect most aspects of your life, including how you think and feel about yourself, your social and work relationships, and your family, it makes sense that asthma can impact your sex life as well. As the saying goes, ninety percent of sex is in the head, and we find that many sexual problems encountered by people with asthma are indeed psychological.

That is not to say that asthma never requires physical changes in the way you make love. If your asthma is mild, however, no physical changes are likely necessary. If you have moderate to severe asthma, some changes in your lovemaking may be helpful. If you are in the group for which some change is required, we're happy to report that in the great majority of cases the solutions are simple. This important part of your life certainly can remain intact.

THE IMPORTANCE OF COMMUNICATION

While it may be relatively easy to talk about problems at work, or changes in the family, it can be difficult to talk about sex. It is just as important to talk with your partner about sex as about shifting roles, responsibilities, and relationships. If your asthma *is* causing sexual problems for you and your partner, not talking about it may not be just part of the problem but the problem itself. Once you begin communicating, some couples find, you really may have nothing to worry about at all. For example, Nate and Jeanette had a normal sex life until Nate's asthma worsened in his mid-forties. That's when they discovered they needed to change just one thing: talking about sex.

    ॐ Nate and Jeanette have been married for almost fifteen years. Nate has had asthma since childhood but never required more than occasional over-the-counter medication until recently, when his breathing began to require regular use of prescription medications. Nate used to say of his sexual relationship with Jeanette, "We don't talk about it; we just do it." And they did, fairly regularly, sometimes spontaneously, and with a large degree of mutual satisfaction.

    When Nate's asthma worsened, so did their sex life. The frequency of their lovemaking dropped from about once a week to once a month, and the enjoyment seemed to diminish for each of them. After about six months, their twelve-year-old daughter came home from school one day and told them about her assignment to practice "active listening," a communication skill in which each person listens to the other and makes sure he or she understands what was said. This communication device turned out to be all that Nate and Jeanette needed to get their sex life back on track.

Active Listening Is Easy

Nate's philosophy—"We don't talk about it; we just do it"—worked well enough before his asthma worsened but not afterward. Nate and Jeanette made the most common mistake encountered by asthma patients when things are not going well sexually; they did not communicate openly about what was happening for *each of them.*

    Open communication is the key to most sexual difficulties that result from asthma. In fact, it is not an exaggeration to say that better communication will go a long way toward solving most relationship problems between people who truly care about each other. And, as a twelve-year-old can tell you, active listening is the key to good communication. Fortunately, active listening is also very easy to do.

When *either* partner decides there is something important to talk over, the couple should set aside a time and place for the discussion. This does not mean during commercials of your favorite television show! Pick a time when you can relax together and listen to each other, free of other distractions. In most families with children this means after the children have gone to bed or are at least well occupied. For couples without children, try active listening over a nice meal, especially on the weekend when you are both feeling refreshed.

The next step is to "lighten up." Serious discussions do not have to be deadly serious. Be easy with each other and yourself, and do not expect to solve all your current communication problems in one sitting. Relax and get ready to listen.

The Problem

The person who called for the discussion should usually go first. Let's assume that's you. It's easy.

1. As clearly as possible, state what you've been feeling, what's concerning you, and what you would like to see changed. Save ideas for possible solutions for later in the talk or for a later date altogether.
2. Then have your partner *restate your thoughts and feelings as your partner heard and understood them.* Your partner should not simply parrot back the exact words (that may feel like sarcasm), but rather *state how he or she understood what you said.* Then your partner asks you if that understanding was correct.
3. If not, you must try again. Use different words this time, try a different approach, but keep trying until your partner really understands what you've said.

4. Once that is accomplished, switch roles and repeat the process with your partner making the opening statement.
5. Keep at it until each person understands what the other thinks and feels about the situation.

This process alone may go a long way toward solving the dilemma.

The Solution

Once the two points of view are well understood, take a break and set a time to discuss possible solutions. Or, if you both feel ready, launch right in. For the solution phase, follow the same format:

1. "This is what I think we can do about it." Don't blame your partner for what has gone wrong; instead, focus on some possible solutions for what needs to be fixed.
2. Have those possible solutions restated and understood.
3. Now come your partner's ideas for problem solving.

Be flexible, compromise, try different solutions, and discuss how they are working. These measures will soon have most problems solved. Just the act of trying to understand the other person's thoughts, feelings, and possible solutions will soften the edges on the most difficult dilemma. Remember to lighten up; most discussions will go better in an upbeat, playful atmosphere. If things get too tense, call a halt and try again later.

Nate and Jeanette's first attempts went quite well.

&⇜ The day his daughter introduced them to active listening, Nate decided to take a risk with Jeanette. He suggested they try active listening about their sex life, and Jeanette readily agreed. They decided to try that evening in the privacy of Nate's study, when their daughter was safely working in her room.

Because Nate had been the one to bring it up, he went first. He told Jeanette that he had noticed the change in their pattern of lovemaking and was unhappy about it. He told her he was worried that she was unhappy with him because he wheezed almost every day and hadn't been helping with the chores as frequently. Jeanette restated her understanding: "You think I'm disappointed in you because your asthma has gotten worse. And you're worried I'm mad at you." Almost before Nate could nod his assent, Jeanette went on, "Oh, Nate, it's not like that at all. I was afraid sex might be hard on your breathing, so I've just been waiting until you took the initiative. I'm not disappointed or mad; I was just worried about you."

It didn't take Nate and Jeanette long to realize what had been happening; both had been holding back because of what they *thought* was happening in the other person, and both had been wrong. That very evening, Nate and Jeanette moved into the next phase of their experiment with active listening. They tried out a solution together!

Whose Anger Is It—Yours or Your Partner's?

The case of Nate and Jeanette illustrates a number of other difficulties often encountered by people with asthma regarding their sex lives. Aside from the obvious problem, that they did not communicate openly about sex, Nate was likely undergoing some emotional reactions to his worsening asthma, and so was Jeanette. These changes may have been affecting their sexual relationship without their knowing it. For example, Nate assumed that Jeanette was angry with him about his asthma. This may have been true, but it is just as likely that *Nate* was angry about his asthma but had not acknowledged it either to himself or to his wife.

Asthma in just one partner is likely to leave both people feeling some anger. And it is very difficult to feel sexy when you are feeling angry. After the problem of not communicating openly about sex, unexpressed or unacknowledged anger is the second most common impediment to a good sexual relationship. Nate was probably angry that his body no longer worked as well as he wished. He may have felt angry at himself for having asthma in the first place, angry at his medications, at his doctors, angry that he could not live the medically carefree lifestyle that he had enjoyed for most of his life. Nate may even have been a bit angry at Jeanette just because he had asthma and she did not. Such reactions to asthma do not make Nate a terrible person or even very unusual.

There is nothing wrong with being angry. It is a normal reaction to any kind of loss, including loss of physical health or freedom. The problem that Nate ran into was that *he was not aware of his own anger*. He thought it was Jeanette who was angry! Because Nate experienced his anger as coming from Jeanette, it made sense that he would hold back from initiating sex. After all, someone who is angry with you is not very likely to want to make love with you, so why not just wait until he or she is no longer mad? Waiting was not going to solve this problem, however, because it was *Nate's own anger* that he was not aware of, *not Jeanette's*.

It is also true that Jeanette may have been experiencing some annoyance at Nate for his worsening asthma. She did need to do more chores, and his general mood was more irritable than before his asthma began to worsen. As we discussed in Chapter 6, their family roles may have needed some adaptation, something the couple had not yet addressed directly. If Jeanette was angry, it would also be important for her to acknowledge it and then attempt to clear the air with active listening and problem solving. It does no good for them to deny their feelings or experience those feelings as occurring only in their partner. A good relationship, sexual or otherwise, depends on openness about one's own feelings.

For a satisfying sexual relationship, both partners must be aware of their own feelings, whatever they are. *Don't let your partner do the feeling for you.* It will only lead to confusion and unclear communication, and your sexual relationship may suffer as a result. Acknowledge your feelings to yourself, communicate them directly to your partner, and problem-solve actively.

Whose Sadness Is It?

In addition to the anger that Nate experienced about his asthma, he felt sadness and loss. Nate worried that Jeanette thought he was "not the man I used to be." As with his anger, it was primarily *Nate*, not Jeanette, who felt that he wasn't the same person he used to be. Asthma may bring on a host of feelings, all grouped under the term *depression*. You may have experienced weight gain from medication use or less vigorous exercise, and as a result you may feel sexually unattractive. You may feel that you are less of a contributor around the home or at work. In general, asthma may leave people feeling less good about themselves and their bodies. In Chapters 2–4, we discussed some ways to cope with these feelings. It is important to remember that how you feel emotionally will impact how you feel sexually. If you feel depressed because of changes in how you view yourself, you are less likely to feel sexual. Don't attempt to deny your sadness or view it as coming from your partner. Neither should you exaggerate it or its impact on your self-worth. Acknowledge the feelings of sadness and loss, but keep them in perspective. Then, set about the work of resolving them in the manner we suggested in Chapter 3.

Work on the Feelings, and the Sex Will Follow

Nate's philosophy of sex without communication was gradually shifted to one of communication first and sex later. This may be an important shift for you and your partner to consider as well. If your emotional reactions to asthma are interfering with your relationship, it's probably best to clear the air first, before those feelings find their way into your sexual relationship. Don't attempt to use your sexual relationship as the means of resolving your emotional dilemmas. Try the techniques we suggest for solving emotional problems first, and many of the sexual problems will disappear. Once you have worked on emotional openness with yourself and your partner, and have worked within yourself on feelings of sadness and anger, if sexual problems persist, they are likely physical, not emotional.

"I'M TOO SHORT OF BREATH TO MAKE LOVE."

So far, this chapter has focused on the emotional pitfalls that asthma patients may encounter in the area of sex. Sometimes, however, it *is* the physical aspects of sex that are the problem.

As with the emotional dilemmas just described, there is no reason to throw up your hands and conclude that relatively severe asthma precludes a normal sex life. Emma knows better:

> ᏭᏉ Emma, a twenty-year-old college student, has had a steady boy-friend for the last year. Most aspects of their relationship have been good, but the sex part was not so good. Emma liked the idea of sex, but she didn't like the act itself. No, Emma did not have some psychological hang-up that caused her to shy away from sex; rather, her asthma was triggered by most forms of physical exertion, including making love. Emma usually found that making love caused her to feel frighteningly short of breath, and so she stayed away from it whenever possible. She used to tell her boyfriend, "I'm too short of breath to make love."
>
> One day, Emma's older sister showed her some materials from a class for pregnant women. Included in the materials was a description of ways to make love that required less physical energy. "That's what I need," thought Emma, and in truth, it was. Emma did not need to avoid sex; she just needed to try some different ways of having sex that would not leave her so short of breath. As it turned out, the next time Emma was in a position to be sexual with her boyfriend, she suggested one of the ways she had discovered. "We curled up together, side by side, with Tommy lying behind me. It felt great, and not just the intercourse part; the holding was nice too."

Emma thought that her asthma made her too short of breath to make love, but all she needed was a willingness to try some new ways of making love. If you can walk up two flights of stairs, you probably have enough physical energy to have a satisfying sexual encounter. You don't need to be able to walk up the stairs quickly. Pacing yourself is good advice in most areas of life, whether walking up stairs or making love. In addition to pacing yourself, your asthma may require that you pretreat with inhaled medications before walking up stairs. The same is true for making love or any other form of physical activity. Don't give up the activity altogether; figure out what you need to sustain the physical demands of lovemaking and then structure your lovemaking accordingly.

Structuring your lovemaking may not sound very romantic,

and we are not recommending you leave the romance out of your sex life. Especially for couples who have been together for some time, the romance, the holding, the caressing may be every bit as important as the sexual intercourse. But we do want you to remember that making love requires physical exertion, and like most forms of physical activity, the more you practice and prepare, the better you get. In fact, preparation is the first step in the three P's of making love for a person with asthma: *prepare, position,* and *play.*

Prepare

You would not expect yourself to run a marathon without adequate training, and the same is true for making love. The preparation stage of making love occurs when your partner is not even present. As we will discuss in Chapter 10, there are a number of ways you can prepare for most strenuous activities. Proper diet and adequate exercise will help ensure that whatever trouble you have breathing is really the result of reactive airways and not an underactive lifestyle. You may be surprised what taking a good walk every day will do for your sex life. Also, as with other forms of exercise, you may need to pretreat with inhaled medication shortly before your lovemaking.

Exercise and diet will help you prepare for lovemaking, and you may discover other things you can do that are more specific to the sex act itself. For example, self-stimulation (masturbation), either alone or when your partner is present, is a good way to prepare for making love with your partner. Through masturbation you can learn what feels good to you, and later you can communicate that directly to your partner. Also, pay attention to your fantasies while masturbating for clues about what you find sexy, and when appropriate, communicate these to your partner as well.

Talk to your partner about what feels good when masturbating? Discuss sexual fantasies? Is it really okay to do these things? Not only is it okay, but also it will almost certainly enhance sexual enjoyment for both of you. If you're uncertain, just ask yourself these questions: Would I like it if my partner told me what felt good to him [her] and then I was able to do it? Would I like to hear some of my partner's fantasies about sex and even try some of them out? If your answer is no, you're probably not yet at the stage of communication with your partner where it is appropriate to discuss such feelings and ideas. If, however, your answer is yes, it's a good bet your partner feels similarly. As long as you communicate openly about your feelings without expecting your partner to do anything more than listen, you should be on safe ground. You really have very little to lose.

Position

In the real estate field there is a saying that success depends upon three things: location, location, location. For an asthmatic person who is experiencing shortness of breath during sex, a similar adage applies. Success depends heavily on position, position, position. The physical positioning of the two partners can be crucial in managing your asthma during lovemaking. Only you can determine what position works best for you and your mate, or if this kind of positioning is necessary at all. If it is, you and your partner can experiment with a variety of positions, some of which are described here. The most important aspect of positioning is to allow the nonasthmatic partner to come to the asthmatic partner. In other words, find sexual positions in which one person is relatively physically quiet, with more physical effort exerted by the other. Have the asthmatic partner assume the more quiet position. If both partners have asthma, have the partner whose breathing is better at the time assume the more strenuous position.

Some of the positions that may be helpful in minimizing physical effort during sex include the following:

1. ***Spooning:*** This is the position used by Emma and Tommy. In this position the man and woman both lie on their sides with the man behind. Intercourse occurs when the man enters the woman from behind. Face-to-face kissing

is difficult in this position, but the man is easily able to caress the woman's body during lovemaking.

2. **Front to front:** In this position the partners lie on their sides facing each other. Frontal touching of both partners is possible, as well as face-to-face kissing. For intercourse, the woman places her upper leg over the man's upper leg. This is an especially good position when both partners have asthma.

3. **Woman on top:** This position is useful when it is the man who has problems with breathing. The man lies on his back in a comfortable position, and the woman sits facing him, legs spread to achieve intercourse. The woman may find this position quite strenuous. If so, after penetration, she may slide down the man's body so that some of her weight is supported by his torso and not just her arms and knees.

4. **Woman kneeling, man behind:** In this position the woman kneels with her back to the man. She may support her upper body with pillows or by kneeling at the foot of the bed with her torso resting on the bed itself. The man, also on his knees, enters the woman from behind and is able to caress her back and front torso during intercourse.

These four positions are only suggestions. Try these and find others that work for you and your partner. Play with different ideas and different positions. *Play*, in fact, is the last of the three P's of lovemaking for an asthmatic person. And it is the easiest of all.

Play

Sex is not work. Yes, it does take a certain amount of concentration and effort, but of a different type than encountered by most of us at work. Be playful during your lovemaking. Lighten up. Play before, during, and after sex. Play with your fantasies and your partner's. Be playful with yourself and with your partner. Play with different positions. Play with sex, and it will require less energy and allow you to breathe easier. Sports psychologists tell us that sometimes the only difference between world-class athletes such as sprinters lies in which one is having more fun, which one is more relaxed during the race. In other words, the successful athlete is the one who plays during the race, not just works hard. The more you play during sex, the easier on your breathing it will be, and the more fun as well!

৵ Chapter 8

How to Live with an Asthmatic Child

One more factor in family adaptation to asthma must be considered: children who have asthma. The chances that your children will have asthma range from twenty-five to sixty percent, depending on whether one or both parents have the disease. As you can imagine, a child with asthma not only adds new twists to the process of family adaptation but personally faces psychosocial challenges not faced by adults. This chapter offers some insight into what your child and your family might encounter if the child develops asthma.

We hope, though, that you will read this chapter even if children do not seem to be in your foreseeable future. Any problems you have coping with asthma today may very well have originated with how your own parents dealt with particular problems posed by your asthma. Sometimes what stubbornly stands in the way of your living well with asthma as an adult is the faulty beliefs entrenched since childhood. As you read through this chapter, ask yourself if the information presented reveals any flaws in your long-held perceptions about asthma. Could your social or emotional development have been impeded by your family's (probably well-intended) attempts to cope with the disorder? The following pages might stimulate the insight you need to solve any remaining adaptation problems of your own. And if you do someday have children, your new self-knowledge can help you keep faulty beliefs out of your children's adaptation to the disease.

We've been concentrating on family adaptation, so let's begin with the impact a child with asthma can have on the whole family.

THE IMPACT OF A CHILD'S ASTHMA ON THE FAMILY

ह≥ "We've had good reason to be worried about Tony," his father commented. "He's needed to be hospitalized seven times in the last two years and was on a respirator during his last hospitalization. We knew Tony's asthma was severe from a very early age and did everything possible to protect him. Seven years ago, when he was five, we arranged our work schedules so that one of us was home with Tony at all times. My wife worked from 6:00 A.M. to 2:30 P.M. I worked from 3:00 P.M. to 11:00 P.M. Now, I never see my wife. We have only one day off in common. There is no way I can discuss things with her. I have more of a relationship with my kids because at least I see them on my day off and in the morning before they go to school."

Tony's parents had made extreme sacrifices in Tony's behalf. They sacrificed their marriage and their family life to be available to him at all times. They had a very poor relationship. When they were together, they had numerous arguments because of the dissatisfaction they felt with their lives. This created a circular situation: the more they fought, the more they wanted to avoid each other; the more they avoided each other, the worse their relationship became. This conflictual home life made Tony's asthma, which was partially emotionally triggered, even worse. The steps Tony's family took were a maladaptive, rather than an adaptive, adjustment to his asthma.

It's very difficult to construct a plan that will address the need to protect your child and the needs of the family. But for the asthmatic child and family, it's crucial. Asthma should never be permitted to ruin family life the way it has with Tony's family. Asthma should not be the central focus of a family—rather, the family itself should be central, with an asthmatic family member being one of the challenges to which the family adapts.

For example, Tony's parents could make certain his school and child-care providers know the appropriate steps to take if Tony has an asthma attack. Parents could provide phone numbers where they can be reached while away. Emergency numbers for friends or family members who are familiar with the child's asthma and the child's doctor could also be made available. One mother, whose child's asthma was very severe, and who traveled on her job, rented a pager so she could be available at all times.

≥ "Janie was so sick as an infant that I gave her lots of attention," her mother, Marie, explained. "When Janie had to be hospitalized, it was always I rather than my husband, Bill, who stayed with her at night. I read about asthma and knew all of the things I needed to do for Janie. Bill left it all up to me and learned little about asthma. This created a very strong and special bond between Janie and me."

"I remember feeling like a fifth wheel," Bill recalled. "I guess, since I felt I wasn't wanted, I became more withdrawn."

"I could feel Bill's withdrawal, but I didn't understand it," Marie explained. "I felt hurt and lonely, so I put even more energy into my relationship with Janie, which was much more fulfilling."

"We were arguing all the time," Bill continued, "and almost always the arguments focused on Janie. I thought Marie babied Janie too much. Marie said I ignored Janie completely, so she had to make up for it."

"I didn't know what to do," Marie complained. "I felt like I was losing my husband, but if I didn't attend to Janie, I might have really lost her."

Healthy families have as their heads two strong parents who communicate and come to an agreement (however hard-won) on childrearing issues. They present a united front to the child. One-parent families can also be of the healthy type if the parent takes a leadership role and is consistent. In Janie's family the main unit was a parent–child one rather than a parent–parent one. This nearly always causes problems.

It's very easy to see how having a child with asthma can have an impact on a couple's relationship. It's very important, however, to put a lot of energy into keeping this relationship strong. Having a child with asthma can be a demanding experience, and the couple will need each other to cope. One way to develop a strong couple and parental bond is to have both parents involved in caring for the asthmatic child. Both should be aware of medications, nebulizer function, and asthma protocols. It's also helpful if they share their fears for the child with each other. This type of behavior can promote good family functioning and emotionally well-adjusted children.

Problems with siblings can also be difficult for a family to manage. Having an asthmatic sibling can create a great deal of jealousy and other problems because asthmatic children can be very demanding. One father remarked:

૎ "Brent [their fifteen-year-old son with asthma] takes up more of our time and energy than our other three children put together!"

It's crucial that other siblings in the family get the attention and quality time with a parent that they need. This may be especially difficult while an asthmatic child is hospitalized, but it is still very important. Siblings should have the opportunity to discuss their worries or concerns about the asthmatic child as well as their jealous feelings. Creating special time with each child to encourage the child's unique characteristics can help all the children in the family feel special and valued. Spending this type of time with each child also helps the child with asthma understand that he or she does not need to be sick to get the parents' attention and love.

Changes in Family Lifestyle

Often, few changes will need to be made in lifestyle, but sometimes your doctor may recommend measures ranging from getting rid of carpets or pets to avoiding vacations in isolated places to—in extreme cases—relocating. These may be painful adaptations, and it may be difficult to make them without feeling resentful of the asthmatic child, especially if the change is giving up a well-loved family pet. In these cases, it's often helpful to discuss the issue as a family and to explore alternatives.

For example, one family found an alternative to giving away their cat. They decided simply to make it an outdoor rather than an indoor cat. The cat was allowed to come into the garage at night, and all the children except the child with asthma could have sleepovers with the cat in the garage. Because the child with asthma could no longer have contact with the family pet, he was allowed to have a choice of pet (to which he was not allergic) to keep in his room.

Another family, who lived in a rural community sixty-five miles from medical care, decided it was worth it to move nearer the city because their child required frequent emergency room visits. In this case, advantages and disadvantages of the move were made the subject of family discussions long before the decision to move was made.

In both cases, the asthma was discussed as a family problem into which everyone had input, although it was ultimately the parents' decision. In Chapter 6, we discussed in greater detail family changes that may be necessary, as well as a step-by-step method for attempting to work on those family problems.

With support, Tony's parents began to rearrange their lives. Tony's father changed to the day shift so he could work from 8:00 A.M. to 5:00 P.M. This enabled him to help the children get off to school and his wife to be available after school. They joined a support group for families with asthmatic children and a baby-sitting co-op with the parents in the group. They made a point of going out as a couple at least one evening a week. They had a number of problems to work out between them at first but gradually became closer and formed a stronger parental unit for the children. While Tony's asthma continued to be severe, they seemed to worry about it less because they knew that they had taken the steps necessary to ensure his safety. Tony described the changes in his family:

ঌ "It's just more peaceful and less tense at home. Mom and Dad don't fight as much, and we've been doing more together. Last week we went camping, and this week we're having a big picnic with friends."

To the benefit of the whole family, Tony's parents solved the problems that had developed between them. They may have been able to nip them in the bud, however, if they had examined some of the beliefs that caused the problems as soon as the damage became evident. For example, Tony's parents were operating on the belief that only *they* could protect their son at all times. To us outsiders, emotionally uninvolved as we are, the flaw in that belief is obvious. And that is one of the biggest hazards for parents of asthmatic children: you *are* emotionally involved. So much so, in fact, that your vision of the truth may become blurred—by love, by your fears for your child, by your deep need to protect your son or daughter. Therefore, it's paramount that you balance your emotions with fear-taming fact. The rest of this chapter offers a few tips for putting yourself through a reality check when needed. Are your decisions regarding your child based as much on reason as on emotion? Do you have a realistic perception of your child's abilities and limitations? Are you prepared to anticipate the new ways that asthma may affect your child at each developmental stage?

YOUR ROLE IN YOUR CHILD'S ADAPTATION TO ASTHMA

Childhood is a time of great physical, social, and emotional development. Asthma can present obstacles to that development if healthy adaptations are not made. As a parent, you have significant control over your child's adaptation.

Elizabeth talks about the problems she had with her daughter Amy, who has severe asthma.

❧ "Before we sought help, my nine-year-old daughter, Amy, was much too dependent on me," Elizabeth confessed. "I just didn't know what to do about it. I felt I had to be near her because she was likely to have an asthma attack and need me to act quickly. At the worst point, she had become so clingy she didn't want to go to school. Amy said she needed to stay home because of her asthma, but I knew it wasn't bad enough to justify her frequent absences. I felt so caught, because I understood her fear of being away from me, and, to some degree, I shared it. I knew it was unrealistic, but I kept thinking that if I watched over her at all times, she would never have a fatal asthma attack. Thank goodness, the physician, nurses, and psychosocial staff at the clinic helped me see what I was doing and how Amy and I could stop the pattern safely. Amy is now much more independent and is going to school regularly. I now feel confident that she will be able to manage most situations should she have an asthma attack."

The dilemma Elizabeth faced is a common one among parents of children who have asthma. Having an asthmatic child, especially if the asthma is severe, can be very frightening. Many children, unlike adults, cannot be relied on to automatically act responsibly in the face of an asthma attack. For children, especially young children, the inability to breathe can be terrifying. At a very early age they understand that their survival depends on the appropriate actions of an adult, usually their mother or father. At times, this can cause a child to become clingy or develop an unusually strong need to be close. Parents of asthmatic children understand this, too, and often make certain they are very available to their children. The fear of having their child die can set up a pattern of extreme caution that can unintentionally interfere with their child's development. Gregory's parents are a good example:

❧ Eleven-year-old Gregory complained of his parents, "They never let me do anything! This is the second time this summer they haven't let me sleep over at Matt's house. They won't let me go to Boy Scout camp and won't let me join the baseball team. My friends are going to stop inviting me places because I never get to do anything." To his parents, Greg pleaded, "Can't I stay over at Matt's house just this once?"

"I don't know what to do," Greg's mother complained.

"Greg's asthma is always worse at night. What if he had an asthma attack at Matt's? I wouldn't be there to help. Matt wouldn't know what to do, and neither would his parents."

Amy's previous need to be near her mother and Greg's parents' need to be readily available to their son interfered with the social and emotional development of both children. Amy's extreme dependence on her mother made it difficult for her to mature. She started to get poor grades and became uncomfortable around her peers because she spent more time with her mother and other adults who protected her than children. Greg will continually get the message from his parents that he is less capable—and has deficiencies that limit his options in life. This can impact the way Greg feels about himself and lead to poor self-esteem. It also can influence his striving to be a mature, independent adult if he repeatedly gets the message he can't make it on his own without close, adult supervision.

Parents want what is best for their child, so many feel trapped by the dilemma of trying to be appropriately protective without impeding the asthmatic child's social and emotional development. Clearly, raising a child with moderate to severe asthma is a difficult challenge. It is possible, however, if a family makes a healthy adaptation to the asthma rather than allowing the fear of asthma to control their lives.

What Is a Parent to Do?

One principle that has helped some parents raise an asthmatic child to become an emotionally healthy and productive adult is attempting to create an optimally average atmosphere. This means attempting to adopt a lifestyle that would exist if the child did not have asthma. This does not mean denying the illness but rather adapting to it in such a way that it will not interfere with the child's development.

This can be accomplished via several steps:

1. Replace fear with realistic decision making.
2. Educate the child about asthma and asthma self-care.

3. Develop a resource base of people who can be relied on to take appropriate steps during an asthma episode.
4. Have enough understanding of developmental tasks at each age to help your child achieve these milestones.

Replace Fear with Realistic Decision Making

Sometimes, as with Greg's parents, fear of the child's dying or having severe asthma attacks controls the parents' decision making. Greg's parents say no every time one of Greg's requests triggers a fantasy of an asthma problem. The first step, then, is understanding and controlling your fear if your child's request is reasonable. If Greg's asthma is unquestionably triggered by grass, camping out in a tent on the grass without adult supervision is not wise. If, however, Greg will be sleeping in the house, and he has been taught appropriate self-care steps, there should not be a problem. *In all cases the child's doctor should guide parents about what activities should and should not be allowed.* Ask your doctor if you can schedule a time to talk and ask questions. Your doctor may be able to give you guidelines (peak flow values, etc.) that you can use along with your experience with your child's triggers to judge whether your child should be permitted to participate in an activity. The same guidelines can also be helpful in deciding whether your child is well enough to attend school.

Here is a series of reality-check questions that parents often find helpful with decision making:

1. Is the activity very likely to trigger my child's asthma?
2. If so, can steps be taken to modify the activity or my child's response to it, so that it is less of a risk?

With Greg, these steps might include (a) allowing Greg to sleep out in a tent if it has a heavy floor pad and is placed on the patio away from grassy areas, and (b) allowing Greg to join the baseball team but having him pretreat before the workouts so as not to trigger his exercise-induced asthma.

3. What is my child's current medical status (experiencing chest tightness, wheezing, clear breathing)?
4. Can my child responsibly take appropriate steps if he or she experiences problems?
5. If not, will there be a responsible adult around who could take appropriate steps?
6. If my child did not have asthma, would I allow him or her to participate in the activity?

Your goal should be to take the necessary steps to prevent asthma problems without being overly restrictive. These questions can also bring you back to earth if you have the opposite tendency, to attempt to compensate for the child's asthma by being either overly permissive or overly generous. A common complaint of siblings of asthmatic children is "He always gets toys he asks for, especially when he's sick or in the hospital. People are always buying him things. Mom and Dad spend so much time with him that I never get any attention. Sometimes it makes me wish I had asthma." Of course, it is difficult not to cater to a sick child, but in the long run giving too much attention and overly extravagant gifts can be problematic. Again, in this case, creating an optimally average atmosphere is a helpful goal.

Educate the Child about Asthma and Self-Care

Understanding what is going on in their bodies helps kids with asthma assuage their fears and take the necessary steps to control their symptoms. Many good books that explain asthma to the child are available; see the Appendix. If you have asthma, you know that asthma has the potential to be a lifelong disease. You'll do your children a great service if you help them learn now to manage it independently and avoid overdependence on you. The following guide, based loosely on the program used at National Jewish Medical and Research Center, will give you a general idea of what level of self-care you can expect from your children according to their age. You will, of course, need to adjust the expectations to match your child's developmental, responsibility, and compliance levels.

Ages Five through Eight:

Children in this age group should be able to:

- Take medications when parents administer them.
- Use good inhaler and nebulizer technique (with careful demonstrations by your doctor).
- Be able to identify and report wheezing to parents.

Ages Eight through Ten:

Children in this age group should be able to meet all the expectations of the earlier age group and:

- Identify asthma triggers.
- Identify early warning signs.
- Properly use a peak flow meter and ask parents to record the value.

Ages Eleven through Twelve:

Children in this age group should be able to meet all the expectations of the earlier age groups and:

- Know the steps to take if they begin wheezing. (This may include a first step of relaxation and deep, slow breathing using the diaphragm, with a second step of using an inhaler if the first step fails; your doctor should be your guide in developing a "wheeze plan.")
- Record and chart daily peak flow values.

Ages Thirteen through Sixteen:

Children in this age group should be able to meet all the expectations of the earlier age groups and:

- Begin to make good decisions about activity participation based on peak flow charts, present respiratory activities, and triggers.
- Self-administer medication with minimal parental super-

vision. (Some parents buy medication reminder boxes and supervise their adolescent while they fill the pill boxes. The parents then need only check the box each day to ensure that the adolescent took the medication.)

Ages Seventeen through Eighteen:

Children in this age group should be able to meet all the expectations of the earlier age groups and:

- Fill medication reminder boxes without supervision.
- Take medication without supervision (although the parent should continue to ensure that medication is being taken).

Develop a Resource Base of People Who Can Help in Emergencies

You'll lead a less worrisome life while addressing the needs of your child if you find several people you can rely on to help care for your child in the event of an asthma exacerbation. The following measures should ease your fears about not being present during your child's every episode.

1. Educating the school. When your child begins at a new school, make an appointment with the school nurse to discuss your child's asthma. If your child needs a nebulizer, make certain the school has one. Give the nurse guidelines about when the child should be sent home (per your doctor's instructions), and when you should be called. If your child requires medication during the day, give the nurse these instructions. If your child's school does not have a nurse, schedule a meeting with the child's teacher. Although teachers are unable to do as much as a school nurse, they are likely to be grateful to be told of your child's medical problem and to have clear guidelines (preferably written) about what to do under what conditions. If you pay attention to the asthma at appropriate times, you can forget about it the rest of the time; and you and your child can lead a normal life.

2. Dealing with baby-sitters. It is very common for parents of children with moderate to severe asthma to be reluctant to leave the child with a baby-sitter. Parents' time alone is very important. There are a few options here. One possibility is to find a stable baby-sitter you can train. A second option is to develop a baby-sitting co-op of parents of asthmatic children. Because these parents have the same problem, they can respond appropriately. Because you share the job of watching one another's child, you can relay all the necessary instructions without feeling as if you're burdening them. These parents are more likely to understand your concern. The other benefit is that you may be able to form a support group with these people to talk about problems, to give general support, and to brainstorm about solutions. Many parents have had a relatively easy time starting these groups simply by putting a notice up in their allergist's or general practitioner's office, or by telling their allergist they would like to start a support group/baby-sitting co-op and asking the doctor to let other parents know. This can also be helpful if your child needs to be taken to a hospital in a hurry and you are not readily available.

3. Ensuring a safe social life for your child. Your child is unlikely to have best friends who also have asthma. There may be times when your child will want to go on a major outing or stay overnight at a friend's house. At these times, it is helpful to tell the responsible adult supervising the activity of what will need to be done under certain conditions. Because you already have a written sheet to give teachers, you can give a copy of this to the parent too.

Understand Developmental Tasks: Different Needs at Different Ages

At each age, children face new developmental tasks that lead to healthy social and emotional growth. Asthma can make meeting these developmental demands more difficult because of the precautions necessitated by the disease. Following is a brief description of the developmental needs of children in specific

age groups and the additional problems that may be encountered because of asthma.

Infancy and Toddlerhood (Birth to Age Two and a Half)

This stage is one of great growth in physiological development,
cognitive development, motor skills, and language skills. During
this period the infant moves from being very dependent on
parents to becoming an increasingly independent little individual. With the onset of crawling and walking, the young toddler
is able to wander away from parents and begin to explore his or
her world. Children at this age have a growing sense of themselves and their own free will, which leads to the familiar
"terrible twos." During this stage children discover that their
own thoughts, feelings, and wishes are different from those of
their parents. Thus, they attempt to assert their will to try out
this new independence. This stage is also one in which the child
develops the capacity to trust another human being. The infant's
relationship with the parents will serve as the pattern for all
future relationships. Basic trust develops when the infant's
needs are readily and consistently met by the parents.

A child whose asthma onset begins before the age of two
may have some difficulty developing this age-appropriate independence, and may become somewhat clingy. This happens in
part because of the difficulties asthma presents for the infant.
Just as infants learn to rely on their caretakers to answer their
needs, they rely on the caretaker to help them breathe in the
event of an asthma attack. Asthma attacks are a special case,
however, because both the infant and the parent understand (on
some level) that breathing is essential to life. Thus, physical prox-
imity and the adults' ability to intervene quickly in the event of
an asthma attack become very important. This may inhibit the
normal independence and exploration away from the parent that
begins at this time. It may give the infant or toddler a sense that
the world is a dangerous place when the child is not under the
close supervision of a parent. This can lead to difficulties with
even brief separations and may set the stage for more serious

problems when separations are necessary, such as at school. Parents understandably want to be sure their infants are safe and therefore stay much closer. They may have some difficulty allowing their children to keep some distance. Infants who are very aware of their parents' needs and anxieties may sense the parents' discomfort and perceive that there is danger in separations.

> ⮞ When Angela, the mother of fourteen-month-old Jenny, noticed that her fearful watchfulness of her daughter was discouraging Jenny's attempts to walk, she quickly changed her behavior. Angela was able to reassure herself she could get to Jenny in time, even if she was across the room. She was able to stop hovering over her daughter or moving Jenny closer every time she was out of arms' reach.

In summary, the challenge of this stage is to attend to the child's asthma while allowing the child to explore his or her world, separate, and develop his or her own personality.

Preschool Years (Ages Two and a Half to Five)

Several developmental milestones are attained during this time span. Children achieve control of body functions during toilet training. Verbal and motor skills continue to improve. The child develops more control over emotions with the growth of cognitive and verbal skills. Children become more aware of their bodies and begin to notice similarities and differences between themselves and others. This typically leads to an identification with the same-gender parent. This is frequently the first major exposure to children outside the family, and the child must therefore learn to get along with others socially. Sharing, tolerating others' wishes, and compromising are tasks children of this age are expected to begin to master.

Children with moderate to severe asthma may be delayed in toilet training because of the sense of doubt about issues of bodily control that arise when asthma symptoms are unpredictable and difficult to control. Because of the stress that emergency room visits and hospitalizations create, the child may have a more difficult time developing control over emotions. If the child has become overly dependent on an opposite-sex caretaker, identification with the same-gender parent may be disrupted. Dependence on adults may also interfere with the development of age-appropriate peer relations.

Parents of asthmatic children can help with social and emotional development during this stage by helping children understand that they have control over their bodies in many ways other than the asthma. Encouraging the growth of verbal, motor, and cognitive skills through interesting activities and setting appropriate and consistent limits can aid in the development of emotional and behavioral control. Helping children feel good about their bodies despite the asthma will lead to a better self-concept. Parental involvement of both parents in the child's care and a close bond between the parents will facilitate the child's identification with the same-gender parent.

> ঌ When four-year-old Eric began regularly to urinate in his pants after an asthma attack even though he had been fully toilet trained at age two and a half, his parents had to reassure him in several ways. They reminded him he could control his wetting and worked hard to compliment him on all the coordinated things he could do (throw a ball, run fast, jump high).

Elementary School (Ages Six through Twelve)

Developmental tasks of the elementary-school years focus primarily on activities outside the family—the development of friendships; better control over behavior and emotions; development of a sense of competence in academic, athletic, and interpersonal areas; and the practicing of some degree of independence from the family. Moral development and the capacity for understanding others' feelings improve during this stage.

Children with asthma may have problems at this stage if their illness requires frequent absences from school. Absences can cause problems with friendships and school progress. Even if the child is able to make up course work, the normal process of comparing one's own progress to the progress of classmates (which typically results in a sense of competence and self-confidence) is disrupted. Frequent absences disrupt the growing sense of independence from the family and may encourage an immature reliance on the family. The act of being ill is typically a self-absorbing one. This can, at times, interfere with the development of empathy and morals, which results from interest in others outside the self. Behavioral problems can result if the tasks just cited are not mastered adequately.

Parents of asthmatic children can help with their children's development at this age by encouraging school attendance unless the child *must* stay at home. Encouraging independent extracurricular activities and involvement in athletics will help with the sense of mastery and competence. Parents can also help their child develop healthy self-esteem by realistically complimenting the child in areas of strength and encouraging growth through hard work in more difficult areas.

> ⥌ Nine-year-old Jonathan's parents quickly caught on to his frequent complaints that he was sick and needed to stay home. After they encouraged him to talk about his fears, he was less worried about going to school. His parents were able to be firm about his coming home from school when he was not ill. When he did have to stay home because of his asthma, his parents would invite his friends to come over to play quietly with him.

Junior High (Ages Twelve through Fifteen)

During this difficult stage the young teen must manage the start of puberty, including the development of secondary sexual characteristics, changes in body function, and the handling of intense sexual feelings. The young teen faces the task of accepting this new, seemingly foreign body. This, along with the wish to be of interest to the opposite sex, leads to a reevaluation of the self. Early teens are involved in a dramatic self-appraisal process in which any deficiencies are felt to be extremely painful and terribly obvious. Successful mastery of this stage involves an acceptance of the self that gives the individual a sense of identity apart from family. The wish to be normal but special is very typical of this age group, which makes the teen very susceptible to peer pressure. Acceptance by others aids in the process of accepting the self. A sense of independence from parents begins to grow as the teen takes on the responsibility of managing the new freedom that is characteristic of most junior high schools.

This is the stage at which asthmatic children tend to have the highest incidence of medical noncompliance and problems with asthma symptoms. The wish to be normal and the hatred of bodily imperfections make the asthmatic teenager long to be disease-free. This often results in a denial of the illness and a refusal to take medication. Teens often convince themselves that asthma is no longer a problem. The inability to accept reactive airways as a part of the self can lead to problems with a sense of identity or to poor self-esteem or body concept. The challenge of facing the world with a distorted sense of self can become too great, and the teen can withdraw. At times this withdrawal takes extreme forms, including skipping school, either by being truant or with the excuse of asthma problems.

Parents of an asthmatic adolescent themselves face a difficult task. Raising an adolescent is difficult to manage under the best of conditions. Raising an adolescent with moderate to severe asthma is often a monumental feat. Helping the adolescent understand that everyone has imperfections and aiding in the acceptance of the asthma as a part of life can help with medical compliance without getting into control battles. Exploring the consequences of not taking the medication—illness, missing out on school activities, possible hospitalization—can help the adolescent choose to be more compliant. Adolescents sometimes need adult help in developing a strategy to take the necessary self-care steps while coping with or avoiding feeling embarrassed in front of peers. Aiding the teen in developing an explanation for friends when taking medication or using inhalers can improve compliance. Alternatively, if the teen cannot emotionally handle taking medication in front of friends, finding ways to comply privately with medication regimens may be helpful. In general, however, the more accepting the adolescent is of the asthma and the need for medication, the more accepting peers will be. Encouraging your teen to participate in activities of interest and helping him or her to develop a healthy self-concept will promote age-appropriate socialization.

&> When the parents of twelve-year-old Tammy found she was not using her inhalers at noon and therefore came home wheezing each day, they sat down with her to discuss the problem. She confessed that she hated her friends to ask about her inhalers and was embarrassed to think they felt she had some terrible disease. Her parents empathized but helped her find ways she could tolerate taking her medications without having to explain. They also helped her see that her wheezing was far more likely to draw attention to her asthma than the inhaler did. Although Tammy was unlikely to accept it emotionally, her parents tried to help her feel that the asthma was not a terrible defect.

High School (Ages Fifteen through Eighteen)

The major task of this stage is practicing for adulthood, which requires several developmental steps. The teen must give up the wish to be a child and to be cared for by adults. Typically, the teen struggles with this issue by seesawing between acting ten years old one minute and acting twenty years old the next. The older adolescent begins to accept more and more responsibility. There is a testing of values and beliefs against those of parents and society in general. Testing of the quality of the adolescent's own decision-making process also occurs at this stage. These practice sessions and tests are played out in the well-known adolescent rebellion.

Opposite-sex relationships take on extreme importance for adolescents as they move toward having a family apart from their family of origin. At times they seem preoccupied with boyfriend–girlfriend relations. Managing sexual feelings and sexual behavior can also be an extremely difficult challenge for the adolescent.

Asthmatic adolescents who are overly dependent because of a failure to manage earlier tasks have an extremely difficult time coping with this stage. Exacerbations of asthma and increased school avoidance are typical of adolescents with this problem, because the fear of separation from parents is so overwhelming. These adolescents are likely to be at home rather than with friends during much of their free time and will be reluctant to date. A general avoidance of all developmental tasks of this age may be noted. Adolescents who have not successfully mastered the tasks of childhood, including a sense of competency and adequate separation from the family, may have problems acting increasingly mature and developing the independence and re- sponsibility necessary for the transition into adulthood.

Parents can help older adolescents by helping them explore fears about separation. Giving the adolescent age-appropriate responsibility and having expectations that they will act accord- ingly can also help. Encouraging extracurricular activities of interest, such as clubs or athletics, can move an adolescent in the direction of independence.

A thorough understanding of these tasks and a careful examination of how your child is managing these developmental steps can go a long way toward helping your child make a healthy social and emotional adjustment. It also goes a long way toward controlling the fear that can make parents a child's greatest obstacle in the process of adapting to asthma.

PART IV

LIVING WELL IN THE WIDER WORLD

ɔ Chapter 9

Asthma on the Job

"**W**hat do you do?" is one of the most frequently asked questions in social interaction. As an adult in this society, you are expected to be financially self-supporting or to perform some service that warrants your being supported by others. Usually, having asthma, even rather severe asthma, does not mean you cannot work. However, just as you may need to make changes in family routine, you may need to make some adjustments to your work environment and work relationships to help you function optimally.

Ted, a pharmacist, encountered a common work-related problem stemming from his asthma. A great deal of Ted's identity was tied to his work, and when his asthma interfered, he initially suffered a loss of self-esteem and felt helpless about how to proceed. Ultimately, he found a creative way to solve his dilemma:

ɞ Ted has largely enjoyed his job as a pharmacist for over twenty-five years. He has seen a number of changes in his profession, and he has adapted well to them through a combination of hard work, flexibility, and continuing education. He views his job as an important one, and his regular customers and coworkers value him highly.

For most of Ted's career he has worked nine to five, Monday through Friday, forty hours a week, with occasional evenings or weekends. That was true until Ted's lifelong asthma worsened in his early fifties, sometimes to the point that he missed half or even whole days at work. This presented little difficulty for the pharmacy, because it had adequate on-call coverage, but it was a big problem for Ted. "For twenty-five years I could count on two hands the number of times I've called in sick. Being reliable was something I took pride in, along with being accurate in my work, of course. But now that my asthma is so bad, I'm missing work all the time, and I just feel terrible about it. It's like I've got one foot in the grave, and I'm only fifty-three. Who knows what my coworkers are starting to think? I could even lose my job if this keeps up. It's a mess. Sometimes I feel like if I can't work like I want, maybe I shouldn't work at all."

Quitting work may have been a financial possibility for Ted, but emotionally it would have been a poor choice. It is obvious how important his work was to his self-esteem; to quit prematurely would likely leave him feeling depressed and unfulfilled. It's easy, of course, for an outsider to be objective about that, but even from the inside Ted should have been able to see that an unnecessarily rigid, all-or-nothing approach hardly provided the only solution. Fortunately, he didn't have to count on self-enlightenment. When a young, female pharmacist approached Ted with the idea of job sharing, what seemed like a near-perfect solution was handed to him.

ॐ Cynthia was a recent pharmacy graduate and also pregnant for the first time. She wanted to continue working through most of her pregnancy, and after, but not full time. After discussing their respective needs, Ted and Cynthia agreed that he would work three-fourths time and she would work one-fourth time. In addition, they would remain flexible in their scheduling, so that if Ted's asthma or Cynthia's pregnancy or child presented an unforeseen problem, the other would try to step in and cover. Since they would be sharing one full-time position, there would be no additional cost to the pharmacy, and the two built in some overlapping time each week to keep open their lines of communication about ongoing projects.

Their employer was delighted with the arrangement, and so were they. As Ted put it, "Once we started the job share, I hardly ever missed work, and if I did, Cynthia took over. That was almost like not missing work at all, since she could pick right up where I left off, and vice versa. Now I could do my job, be there most of the time, and if my asthma was particularly bad, the pharmacy didn't miss a beat."

Whether you've been in the workforce for twenty-five years like Ted or you are applying for your first job out of school, many of the same general principles apply. First, assess if and how your asthma impacts your work potential. Second, try to design and implement a plan that makes sense for you and your employer. If your asthma is mild, it probably will not impact your work at all, as long as the physical environment is free of obvious environmental triggers such as solvents, dust, or smoke. And, of course, the level of physical work must be such that it does not trigger an attack. If your asthma is moderate to severe, some accommodations may be required.

If you're just entering the workforce, take honest stock of what impacts your asthma as it might pertain to work:

- Do you react to certain environmental triggers such as dust and smoke, but not to others such as cold temperatures?
- Does physical exertion act as a trigger, and if so, how much can you exert yourself before experiencing difficulties?
- How often do you need a break?
- Does emotional stress easily trigger your asthma?

Once you have these questions answered, look for work that suits you and your asthma. Remember, not only should the physical environment be a good fit, but so too should the emotional environment. For example, if your asthma is very reactive to emotional stress, a job with monthly deadlines may not be best for you. If you're contemplating a job with a difficult physical aspect, try simulating the work requirements at home before committing to the job. Ask your doctor about pretreating before particularly physically demanding parts of the day. Fi-

nally, don't assume that work environments are fixed and unchangeable. Just as we will ask you to be flexible in your
thinking, you may want to see if a prospective employer might
be flexible too. Later in this chapter you will hear from some
employers about what they look for in an employee with
asthma.

BE ACTIVE AND FLEXIBLE

At first, Ted's thinking about asthma and his job was so rigid he
could not think of creative solutions; he got stuck on "work as
usual" or "no work at all." Spurred on by someone else's need
to be flexible, he found a solution that worked for him and his
employer. Ted was lucky because someone else was flexible for
him, but if you need to make changes, don't wait for someone
else. Flexibility is the hallmark of living well with your asthma.

It doesn't matter if you're a pharmacist, teacher, business
executive, or assembly line worker, most people feel less good
about themselves if their asthma requires a change in their
normal work pattern. Loss of work does not mean just loss of
income. It also may result in less social contact, loss of social
status, and lowered self-esteem from feeling less productive.
Feeling less productive can easily lead to feelings of worthless-
ness and, ultimately, to depression. Don't passively give in to
this pattern. As illustrated by Ted, don't be rigid in your thinking
about your job or your own self-worth. In other words, don't be
passive and rigid; be active and flexible.

When we say *be active*, that doesn't mean you should expend
tremendous effort looking for the perfect work environment to
accommodate your asthma. Except in extreme situations, it's
usually better to spend your energy trying to change your
current work environment than to look for a new, perfect one.
For one thing, asthma's impact on your work may continue to
change, and it doesn't make sense to continually look for a new
job. For another, the perfect job is as elusive as the perfect family

(see Chapter 6). Jan, a forty-year-old high school English teacher with asthma, couldn't find a new workplace, but she could change the conditions in the one she had.

&» "The life of a high school teacher is stressful these days," says Jan. "With six classes each day, you take your breaks when you can find them—and where, in my case." Jan's school permitted smoking in part of the teachers' lounge. As far as Jan was concerned, that meant smoking was permitted throughout the entire lounge. "They tried to divide the lounge and filter the air, but, of course, it didn't really work."

Jan knew that well over half of the teachers who used the lounge came there to smoke, so she did not think it was fair to ask to have the policy changed altogether. Instead, she began investigating other schools in the district with a different policy. She found two schools with no-smoking policies, but neither had an opening for an English teacher. She considered a change to teaching civics, but the work involved in starting a new curriculum seemed daunting. "Which to do," she debated, "alienate my friends or work extra-hard myself?"

Jan took her dilemma to the principal. She explained the problem with the room, the filtration system, and the particular problems associated with second-hand smoke and asthma. The principal requested that she make a brief presentation at the next teacher–staff meeting. Aided by some handouts from the American Lung Association, Jan made her presentation, and the group voted to change the policy of the teacher's lounge to make it a no-smoking room.

"I guess I should have started with what I knew best: education."

Ted discovered that his asthma required that he work less and with greater flexibility. Jan, however, needed a change in the work environment itself to accommodate her asthma. She educated her employer and coworkers about asthma, and the environment was made healthier for everyone. It is an interesting coincidence regarding asthma: many of the changes that you may require are actually healthy for most people, not just for people with asthma.

If you cannot work exactly how you want, consider flexible alternatives. An initial consideration should be to work the same schedule but in a work environment that does less to trigger your asthma. There are many work environments that can potentially trigger asthma attacks, and your doctor can help you identify which are the triggers for you. Some of the common work environment triggers to watch for include the following:

- Cleaning solvents, detergents, and bleaches
- Common dust or work-related dusts, such as metal dust
- Fertilizers, plant pollens, and molds
- Fiberglass
- Varnishes, dyes, paints, and resins
- Adhesives and plastics
- Smoke

If your work environment subjects you to one of these triggers, or anything that serves as a trigger for your asthma, first attempt to educate your employer and then alter the work environment. Jan eliminated smoking from the teacher's lounge. Other common solutions are air filters, air conditioners, and masks. It may be possible for your employer to use a different detergent or cleaning solvent, remove plants, clean dust more thoroughly, or make other reasonable accommodations that actually may improve the work environment for everyone.

Some types of work will be more difficult to adapt to your asthma than others. Very strenuous work that needs to be done consistently on a tight schedule may, for example, overtax your breathing capacity. In reality, most perfectly healthy people find this kind of work difficult to perform consistently well. In such situations, changing the type of work you perform regularly may be necessary. In less dramatic examples, however, adapting your schedule, as Ted did, or your work environment, as Jan did, may be all that is required.

You may want to consider a variety of other possible changes depending on your actual medical situation. For example, you may do better working fewer hours per day but stretched over six days per week. Consider working Monday, Tuesday, Thursday, and Friday during the day and part of Wednesday evening to give yourself a midweek break. Some asthmatics work best with regular, brief breaks every couple of hours, with some time then added at the end of the day. If the circumstances of your job cannot be altered sufficiently, lateral moves within an organization to a job better suited to your asthma may be necessary. Finally, you may be able to take advantage of cyberspace. Working with computers at home, or partially at home, is becoming increasingly popular and realistic. Working partially at home is likely to be good for your asthma in terms of the physical environment, the ease of taking breaks, and the relatively low stress level.

EXERCISE YOUR WORKER'S RIGHTS

It did not take Jan much effort to change her work environment once she decided to educate rather than move away. Sometimes, however, you may find that your employer is not so accommodating. When this occurs, you should know that you may have legal rights associated with your health, on both state and federal levels. Consult your state government for the particulars of your state rights. The federal guidelines are described briefly here.

The federal government and most states have laws forbidding discrimination against the handicapped. The concept underlying these laws is that individuals whose physical abilities are impaired should not be deprived of work that they are capable of performing. *Every employee or job applicant should be evaluated on his or her present ability to meet the requirements of the job.* In addition, your employer may be required to make "reasonable accommodation" to the work environment to allow you to perform your work, such as providing a smoke-free environment.

The Employee Retirement Income Security Act of 1974 (ERISA) made it unlawful for an employer to discharge or discriminate against someone's participation in an employee benefit plan. In other words, employers cannot use the potential cost of a medical plan for someone with asthma as reason for firing or not hiring that individual if the person is able to meet the job requirements. The rising cost of health care affects everyone, but if you can do your job without going beyond the guidelines for the use of sick or personal leave, having asthma is not grounds for hiring someone else or dismissing you. Of course, if your asthma is caused by a work-related, occupational exposure of some kind, you may be covered under the workers' compensation laws as well.

Your employer may view hiring someone with asthma as an act of kindness, but don't fall prey to that kind of condescension. If you can do the work you were hired for, do it without apology to your employer or coworkers. You do not owe them anything more than your best efforts as an employee, no more or less than any other employee, with or without asthma.

Be Honest; Don't Be Apologetic

Your sick or personal leave is part of your job's benefit plan. You are entitled to use it when necessary, in accordance with your employer's guidelines. There is nothing to hide or apologize for when making appropriate use of sick leave. After all, you do not feel guilty about having an employee pension plan; why should you feel guilty about using another benefit such as sick leave?

The reasons most people feel uneasy about using sick leave are the wish not to anger an employer and guilt about the extra workload on their coworkers. As we discussed, you are entitled to use the benefits provided by your employer. Recrimination by your employer for the appropriate use of sick leave is improper and probably illegal. For many people, however, guilt about burdening coworkers is of even more concern. Jane is a medical/surgical nurse who was so concerned about overburdening her fellow nurses that she made herself sick!

&ë "I guess I'm a typical nurse," says twenty-eight-year-old Jane. "I give and give until I have nothing left." Despite her asthma, Jane worked the hospital's normal eight-hour day, five days a week. When the hospital shifted nurses' schedules to ten-hour days and reduced some of its staff, the burden increased for everyone. Now, Jane not only worked a ten-hour shift but also was frequently asked to work an extra day every other week. The additional hours took a toll on Jane, and her asthma began to worsen. By the end of each day, she was exhausted, and her breathing was bad, but she pushed on.

Jane's physician suggested that she work only her required forty hours, and if her asthma was bad, she should take sick time for full or even part days to help her maintain a stable breathing pattern. Jane resisted the idea of eliminating extra shifts, and she refused to take sick time for her asthma. "It's not that my supervisor would mind that much; we have pool nurses to fill in, but I know what time off does to the rest of the nurses. They end up working extra hard, because even if a pool nurse is brought in, she can't really pick up all the slack." By the fourth week of her new schedule, Jane was having trouble breathing by noon. After eight weeks, her breathing was poor most of the time. Finally, Jane suffered such a bad attack she needed to leave the floor and was admitted to the hospital. She was an inpatient for three days. After discharge, Jane took her physician's advice. She refused overtime and began to take sick leave when she needed it, usually in small increments. Gradually, her health returned to normal. As Jane put it, "I was so worried about burdening the other nurses, I made myself sick. You don't have to be a nurse to know that's bad medicine."

In addition to being honestly concerned about her coworkers, Jane may have been attempting to overcompensate for her asthma, working extra-hard to prove to herself and others that she was as good a worker as any other nurse, with or without asthma. Try to avoid this temptation. Working with asthma is not about proving yourself; it is about living a normal life, not a superhuman life. You do not have to be better and more hardworking than everyone else because you have asthma. If your asthma requires that you make a change in your typical work routine, the first step is to be honest with yourself. Having some limitations does not mean you're worthless. As we discussed in Chapter 3, such irrational beliefs will only make matters worse and contribute to feelings of depression.

Acknowledging your limits to yourself is the first step; letting your employer know may be the second. Don't attempt to hide your asthma from your employer. There are several reasons for this. First, hiding your asthma implies to yourself that it is something bad, something to be ashamed of, something that cannot be tolerated by others. None of these is true. It is a medical condition, a rather common one, and one that you can adapt to with proper medical and self-care.

A second reason not to hide your asthma is that you may jeopardize your employment if you are not honest about your limitations. Although it is true that you should not be passed over for employment or dismissed because of asthma if you can do the required work, it is also true that employers don't like surprises. Be as open and honest with your employer and coworkers as possible, and you are likely to find they will respond with honesty and respect. In Chapter 4, we discussed Marty, the insurance executive, who hid her asthma from her boss and coworkers. Because she used her inhaler in the bathroom, Marty's boss had started to imagine much worse about her than that she had asthma. When she was honest, her boss was relieved, her coworkers were supportive, and her overall standing not only did not suffer but also may even have increased once people saw her as a hard worker despite her asthma.

THE BOSS'S POINT OF VIEW

Not every employer reacts the same to a worker with asthma, but here is a sampling of those who spoke candidly about their experiences with an asthmatic employee at work. First, the owner of a small printing firm describes his experiences with asthmatic employees:

ও "I don't ask anything more or less from an employee with asthma than any other employee. They need to be honest with me, give me their best effort, and treat their coworkers with respect. I ask that they use their sick time for doctor's appointments, and if they need more time away from the shop, they have to make it up. Once an asthmatic employee asked that I restrict cologne and perfume in the office, and I had no problem with that; I doubt anybody else did either. I guess just honesty and hard work is what I ask, and if they have asthma, diabetes, or anything else, we can try to work with it."

The head of a bottling company said the following:

ও "The only time I ran into trouble with an asthmatic employee at work was once this fellow expected me to know what asthma was, what we needed to do to accommodate it, and so on. Well, I didn't know the first thing about it, but when he told me, I said, 'No problem.' If he wanted to make some of his sales calls from home, it was okay with me as long as he got them done. We even brought in a nurse to talk to at a company meeting once, an educational thing on asthma and some other topics like stress. As long as they let me know what they need, we're okay."

ও "Yeah, I've had experience with an asthmatic employee," replied the head of a large engineering firm. "Turned out they liked things just like I do, clean. So we cleaned the floors and carpets about twice as often. To tell you the truth, I'd been getting a little congested myself, and that seemed to help."

The vice-president of a large clothing maker was less understanding but still helpful.

ও "I don't expect everybody to be the same. Some people can't climb stairs; we've got elevators. Some have trouble hearing; we put amplifiers on their phones. If you've got asthma and you want to stay away from the machine room, no problem. Find something you can do for me and I'll usually let you do it. It's really none of my business, anyway, as long as you pull your weight."

Finally, the head of human relations at a medical billing firm reports:

▸ "Actually, I have many people with asthma. We joke about it here; HCFA [health care] forms on the left drawer, inhalers in the right. It's perfect for them, really—work with computers and phones, take breaks when you want, nice clean environment for the computers and the people. Most I ever had to do was move someone's cubicle because her office vent was too close to a loading dock. She did the right thing; told me right away what the problem was, and an hour later it was fixed."

Not all work-related problems will be fixed so easily, but many can be. *Honesty, flexibility,* and *education* are the words we hear over and over from employers. If you're valuable as an employee, you're probably valuable as an employee with asthma. You might be surprised to hear how infrequently the accommodations suggested by asthmatics were rejected by employers. Typically, the employers just want to understand what is needed, why it is needed, and if there are cost-effective ways of doing what is necessary. Most employers acknowledge that good employees are hard to find and important to keep.

YOUR WORK IS NOT YOUR WORTH

If the suggestions in this chapter are not enough, and you find, for whatever reason, you cannot maintain paid employment at all, it is still very important to find something productive and useful that you can do. In our culture it is easy to equate work, especially paid work, with your worth as an individual. The two are not the same, and you shouldn't fall prey to such narrow-mindedness. It is true, however, that work often provides social contact, support, and status that are important. If you cannot work, try to replace these losses; don't merely accept them as a consequence of your asthma. You may elect to join a service or charitable organization, a book club, or some other social activity. Volunteer your time and abilities to an organization that interests and needs you. Usually, volunteer activities are more flexible, less demanding in general, than paid work. Use this flexibility to your advantage. Volunteer at the library, the schools, your church or synagogue, or anywhere that has a need that matches your interests and abilities. The local United Way is often an excellent resource for finding interesting volunteer activities in your community. Remember, your worth as an individual is not equal to the money you are paid, nor the hours you put in, but rather in your ability to develop your personal potential and make a meaningful contribution to the lives of others.

❧ Chapter 10

A Rich and Rewarding Social Life

Asthma, in moderate and severe forms, can have a profound impact on your social and recreational life if you don't make an adaptive adjustment to the disease. Many times, asthma sufferers give up participating in activities they enjoy either because of asthma exacerbations or out of fears of encountering triggers that may set off a serious asthma episode. Jack tells of the problems he confronted in attempting to make an adaptive adjustment to his problems. He is a forty-year-old man who had mild asthma most of his life. In his late thirties, for unknown reasons, his asthma became more severe.

❧ "I used to play handball with friends two or three times a week. In the last two years, my asthma has become so bad that I would be wheezing after only ten minutes of the game. I started to turn down handball invitations. I didn't realize how important these games were to my life until they were gone. I began to feel like a real invalid and became very depressed. Finally, my wife encouraged me to talk with my doctor about it. He had several useful suggestions, including using my Albuterol inhaler a half hour before a game. He said that if that didn't work, I might consider switching games to something that had longer pauses and required less continuous running, like tennis. Fortunately, the Albuterol did the trick. I play almost as much as I did before. My

172

depression disappeared, and I began to feel like my asthma didn't need to hold me back."

Thanks to the encouragement of Jack's wife, the help of his doctor, and good management techniques, Jack was able to lead the more active lifestyle he desired. Jack had become depressed and withdrawn because of his decreased capacity to exercise. For some people, however, the asthma exacerbations are profound and impact a significant portion of their functioning. This was the case for Maggie, a forty-six-year-old divorced woman with grown children. She had had moderate asthma most of her life, with one severe exacerbation at age thirteen that required a hospitalization. In the last year, however, she had had multiple severe exacerbations.

ತ "Around the time of my divorce, eight years ago, I became much more involved with my church. I served on various committees and found I got a lot of support from other members of the church. My faith and the people in the church became my major sources of emotional support. My whole social life revolved around church activities. In the last year, my asthma has become severe. I have had so many episodes that have required the use of steroids that I resigned from all of the committees I served on. I felt I just couldn't be counted on. People still call, however, and ask me to help with various church activities. I might feel fine on the day they ask me, but I can't predict how I will feel on the day when I am needed. So now when they call, I just say no. I haven't really explained why, because I don't want people feeling sorry for me, and so many people think asthma is 'all in your head.' The more I decline to participate, the more withdrawn and depressed I feel. Other than the infrequent visits from my busy children, I have no social life. Sometimes I think it would be better if the asthma just finished me off."

The extreme depression Maggie feels is understandable given the strategies she has used to deal with her asthma exacerbations. Her feelings of depression and hopelessness are clear signs that she has not successfully adapted to her asthma. Maggie felt stuck with the solution she had chosen because of her strong belief that people would either feel sorry for her or think that it was "all in her head." Eventually, when Maggie's depression became so severe that she had lost her appetite and was not sleeping, she told her physician about the problem. He referred her to a therapist to help with the depression and again reassured her that asthma is a real disease of the lungs.

Once Maggie began therapy, she was able to begin exploring reasons for her depression. With the supportive help of her therapist, using essentially the same process outlined in Chapter 3, she began to examine the perceptions that had led to her strong belief that people would reject her if she told them she had asthma. She recounted that when she was a child her parents had derogatorily spoken about her cousin, Rita, who had asthma. They had talked about how the asthma was "all in Rita's head" and the many ways Rita used the asthma to get out of school and other undesirable activities. Maggie's family actively avoided Rita's family because the family had canceled so many invitations at the last minute due to Rita's asthma. As Maggie began to examine her family's reaction to Rita, she recognized that, despite the surface similarities, there were many differences. Rita was a child who had learned to use her asthma to avoid activities she didn't like. Maggie remembered one year when Rita had attended school for only two months. Maggie was certain that Rita's asthma had not been incapacitating during the other seven months. Maggie also recollected that the problems between the two families were complex and that Rita's asthma may have served as a convenient excuse not to associate.

These revelations were enough to convince Maggie intellectually that her belief that she'd be rejected because of her asthma was faulty. She still, however, did not feel comfortable reviving her social life, so she and her therapist explored further. Eventually, Maggie came to understand that her involvement in her church and her many friendships there had substituted for her ex-husband's presence. The loss of those relationships had rekindled her feelings of loneliness and loss after the divorce. She found that she had never adequately dealt with these feelings.

After Maggie understood and dealt with these issues, the search for solutions came easily. She decided to be honest with her fellow church members about her problem. She told her therapist, "If they are as supportive as I think they are, they will understand if I am ill on the days when I'm needed." Maggie's therapist suggested that she might find a substitute to fill in for her when she was unable to attend. Maggie recognized that she could choose to perform duties that could be done by someone else easily, rather than positions of extreme responsibility, like chairing a committee. Once Maggie began putting some of these suggestions into effect, she began to feel much better.

> "I started back slowly, acting on committees where I knew I would not be missed too much should I become sick. I also explained the situation to a few friends who were also on the committees. I was surprised by the response I got. They had felt my withdrawal was a rejection of them and were relieved when I explained the situation. No one thought the asthma was 'all in my head.' In fact, most people knew someone close to them who has had the disease. I also asked my twenty-one-year-old daughter to substitute if I became ill. Despite her busy schedule, she agreed to help me. I guess she was really concerned about my depression. I also decided to invite some of my friends from church to do other activities with me. I realized I did not need to rely just on church activities for my social life. I feel so much better; I wish I had made the changes earlier."

People with asthma are often tempted to cut out major activities that are vital to their emotional well-being. Some may be afraid that the unpredictability of exacerbations will interfere with plans. Others may fear that the exposure to triggers, including food, animals, smoke, perfume, pollen, grasses, and viruses, will lead to an exacerbation. Although the prevailing wisdom in asthma management is to avoid triggers, even good advice can be taken too far. Turning down all dinner invitations because you might be exposed to a food trigger is extreme. Checking with the host, hostess, or chef to make sure that the dish you have ordered does not contain the offending triggers is not extreme. Likewise, avoiding all shopping because walking past the perfume counter sets off wheezing may be more than is required. Giving perfume counters a wide berth or pretreating before shopping (if avoidance is not possible) will enable you to continue a pleasurable activity.

If you're lucky, you'll have a full and fascinating social life, just like anyone without asthma. And, just like anyone without asthma, you won't be able to predict every detail of every situation you end up in. Life without surprises can be awfully dull, so the best route for us all is to prepare as well as we can for life's hazards and then enjoy the interactions we're fortunate to have with those around us. As an asthmatic person, you'll find this easier to do if you apply the lessons you've learned in the rest of this book:

- *Examine your fears and other emotions for faulty beliefs* that may lurk behind them; see Chapter 3.
- *Communicate with friends and colleagues with whom you'll be spending time.* Tell them about your asthma, tell them what that means you may need from them, and when it feels comfortable, tell them about your doubts and concerns. By now, you probably know, if you've tried open communication with your family and coworkers (see Chapters 6 and 9), that most people will rise to your support if only you give them a chance. Why would friends and associates be any different?
- *Be prepared.* Avoid triggers when you can—again, ask hosts and proprietors what conditions you can expect—and when you must make modifications of your lifestyle, make small ones, one at a time, at a slow pace. Rather than give up your morning jog with friends, find out if any of them would be willing to switch to a walk once or twice a week.
- *Be assertive* (see Chapter 4). There's no need to be an apologist in the social realm any more than in your work world. You have a right to a smoke-free environment, especially if you've called ahead to establish that one is available at a restaurant or other public place. If you need to scale back on commitments to community organizations, say so without shame.
- *Be flexible.* Compromise when you're asking friends to accommodate your asthma, suggest alternatives when you have

to bow out of a commitment, and substitute other attractive activities if you simply must give something up.

• *Be creative.* You may have to use your imagination more than your nonasthmatic friends. How about an old-time ice-cream social at the local ice-cream parlor instead of the traditional potluck supper in the dusty community center? A Scrabble tournament to go along with your club's senior Olympics? You'll find that your creativity blossoms with use, which is especially rewarding when friends start calling you for ideas "because you're so innovative."

• *Do your homework.* Remember, education is the best medicine for your fears of the unknown. You can't foresee everything you'll run into in your social pursuits, but you can certainly keep abreast of any environmental law that affects you, share ideas via a support group, and read, read, read. That brings us to the last, but hardly the least, provision you should take for maintaining a safe and satisfying social life with asthma.

• *Consult your doctor.* In all cases when you have a question about how your asthma will be affected by a particular social activity, it's best to consult your doctor. Your physician may have a good solution. Think creatively and generate all possible ways to continue the activity you love while being prudent in avoiding triggers. Explore these options with your physician. Your physician's advice is irreplaceable in developing strategies for continuing or modifying any desired activity while still acting wisely to avoid an asthma episode. Exercise is one such activity.

DON'T SAY NO TO EXERCISE

There a number of excellent reasons to engage in an exercise program if you have asthma. Being in top physical shape means that you will be better able to tolerate the demands that asthma places on your body. Regular exercise should help compensate for the problems of calcium absorption and brittle bones associated with the use of corticosteroids. People who have previously led a sedentary lifestyle find that a gradual increase in exercise raises the threshold for a bronchospasm (that is, it takes more strenuous exercise to trigger one). Improvements in body image (as discussed in Chapter 3) also tend to improve. In general, people who exercise regularly often report they have more energy, sleep better, and experience less fatigue. In addition, feelings of emotional well-being are reported by many people.

Many people with asthma avoid exercise, perhaps because of the poor response they have had to exercise in the past. In truth, exercise can, in people with exercise-induced bronchospasm, trigger an asthmatic episode. There are many ways around this, however. In fact, many Olympic medal winners have had exercise-induced bronchospasm (forty-one in the 1984 Los Angeles Olympic Games; sixteen in the 1988 Seoul Olympic Games). These people have obviously succeeded in effectively managing their asthma to the point that they are among the world's top athletes. Certainly, if they can accomplish that, it's likely you can continue (or start) an exercise program that you enjoy.

- *If you do not have exercise-induced bronchospasm, consult your doctor about starting an exercise program that is appropriate for the severity of your asthma.*
- *If you know you have exercise-induced asthma but would like to engage in an exercise program, there are two ways to go about it:* (1) with the aid of beta-adrenergic bronchodilators or (2) using a nonpharmacological approach with which your doctor agrees.

Exercise with Bronchodilators

This is a very simple yet effective approach. With your doctor's approval, you use a beta-agonist inhaler (such as Alupent®, Metaprel®, Proventil®, or Ventolin®) twenty or thirty minutes before exercise. In most cases this virtually eliminates all asthma symptoms during exercise.

Exercise without the Use of Medication

This approach is somewhat more difficult to achieve and takes some experimentation but has been used successfully by some individuals. In their book, *Asthma and Exercise*, Nancy Hogshead and Gerald Couzens (in consultation with Dr. Roger M. Katz of the University of California at Los Angeles) outline a step-by-step method: (1) pre-exercise, (2) exercise, and (3) post-exercise. In the pre-exercise phase, there is a period of slow warm-up followed by a rest period. The length of the warm-up period necessary may vary among individuals. Some top athletes can engage in this warm-up period for forty minutes without experiencing a bronchospasm. Some people may experience a "refractory period" in which any chest tightness lessens and they feel as if they can breathe freely. Other people may totally avoid a bronchospasm with this slow warm-up. During the exercise period, breathing is done through the nose or, in cold weather, through a scarf or mask. All of these methods tend to warm and humidify cold, dry air, which is thought to trigger reactive airways. Some athletes use controlled, patterned breathing techniques, which appear to help. During the post-exercise phase, it is very important to cool down slowly rather than stop suddenly. Slow, deep breaths that take air deep into the diaphragm help to prevent bronchospasm. If you can use this approach without experiencing a bronchospasm, you may not need medication. However, if you find that despite the use of these techniques you are still struggling through a bronchospasm until you exercise through it to get to a refractory period, you may need to resort to the use of mediation. Some pulmonary specialists believe that lungs sustain some permanent damage the more they are forced to endure asthma episodes without the aid of pharmacological agents.

Which Exercise Should I Choose?

Try to continue exercises you enjoy with the preceding tips. If these are unsuccessful, switching to an exercise that involves brief bursts of energy sometimes proves helpful. These include doubles tennis, baseball, football, and similar activities that do not require sustained activity over a long period of time. Swimming is believed to be a good exercise for individuals with asthma because the swimmer breathes in the highly humidified air just above the water.

Whatever activities you enjoy, you don't need to say no just because you have asthma. With careful management and creative adaptation techniques, you can continue to live your life to the fullest.

ᔬ Chapter 11

"I Like My Doctor, But . . ."

A good working relationship between you and your doctor is essential to the effective medical and psychosocial management of your asthma. If you and your doctor see yourselves as two individuals teaming together to fight this disease, you'll have a better chance of success than if there are conflicts between you. This is true for most disease processes but seems particularly true in the management of asthma because communication about the feasibility of recommended lifestyle and environmental changes and problems of taking medication at specific times through various delivery systems (oral, inhaler, nebulizer) is so important to effective management. To develop a workable plan, the physician and patient must work together. It is therefore very important that problems that interfere with this process be addressed promptly. Often, patients are happy with many aspects of their physician's treatment but have some specific complaints. Michelle described the problem she had and the way she went about solving it.

ᔞ "I used to leave my doctor's office fuming half of the time," Michelle recalled. "He didn't seem to listen to my concerns or to help me with strategies for dealing with the daily dilemmas I faced in managing my asthma. He was so rushed, he didn't seem to care about me. It got so bad that I had nearly decided to change doctors. The trouble was, he knew my history so well, and my asthma improved considerably under his care. Ultimately, I decided to talk with him about it. At the beginning of an appointment, I told him I had some concerns and asked him if I could speak with him then or if I should schedule a longer appointment the next time. He responded with genuine surprise, and he suggested I come in the following week. I told him what had been bugging me, and he not only apologized but agreed to try to change. Since then, I have been very happy with him. I think I am even more careful to follow his instructions. I am also more careful about not taking up too much of his time."

Michelle actively sought to solve the problem she had with her physician. Unfortunately, many patients who feel the way Michelle did either switch doctors—sometimes several times, and often to the detriment of their physical health—or stay put but carry around an ever-growing burden of resentment and anger. Obviously, those unexpressed emotions will have an impact on how many of their physician's recommendations they are willing to follow.

Michelle's response was exemplary. Because of the positive steps she took, her story has a happy ending. She took a risk and talked with her doctor about her concerns.

INGREDIENTS IN THE DOCTOR–PATIENT RELATIONSHIP

The relationship between a particular doctor and patient is the product of a complex interaction of multiple factors: the individual personalities of doctor and patient, the doctor's specific training and competence, pressures imposed by the medical profession, changing roles of physician and patient (from an autocratic, hierarchical one to a relationship based on collaboration between physician and patient in decision making), patients' expectations of the doctor–patient relationship, and patient attitudes toward the medical profession and medical treatment. A successful relationship depends on the cooperative efforts of both people involved. But even when both are doing their part, influences over which neither has complete control may create problem areas.

Practical Constraints for Physicians

Many pressures on physicians, including time, emotional, and professional constraints, may prevent them from being as responsive to their patients as they might otherwise choose to be. Most physicians feel ethically (and sometimes financially) bound to see all of the patients who need their care. Often, the number of patients that need to be seen in a single day is daunting. This limits the amount of time the physician can spend with each patient. Some physicians have mastered the ability to contain this pressure so that they present a calm, interested demeanor toward the patient. Many physicians do not have this ability. With their often brusque manner, hurried language, and tendency to do two things at once, they communicate that they need to get on with things. Most patients are left feeling that their problem can't possibly be significant. The fact is that most physicians are willing to make time for a patient who has questions or concerns that impact the patient's care—if not at the moment, then at a later consultation time or a longer follow-up appointment.

Emotional constraints impact the physician in ways that may make patients feel unimportant. Doctors deal with many situations daily that are extremely sad, disappointing, or frustrating. Allowing each patient encounter, with all of its accompanying emotions, to fully penetrate would be overwhelming for any human being and would likely negatively impact the physician's functioning. Most medical schools, internships, and residencies encourage a concerned but distant approach with patients. This doesn't mean that your doctor does not care about you. It is likely that your doctor does care but can't feel the emotions you feel to the extent that you feel them. Unfortunately, this stance often comes across as "You don't matter to me; you're just another patient." Because many patients want so much more from their physicians, this is very disappointing and may cause tension between the patient and the doctor.

Professional constraints also place a great deal of pressure on the physician. Not every decision that a physician makes is one of life or death, but some are. What is true of every patient encounter, however, is that a physician must quickly and thoroughly assess all of the essential information, make a rapid diagnosis (or order more tests to help clarify the diagnosis), and develop an appropriate treatment plan—all in a matter of minutes. Because medicine is not an exact science, and each patient's physiology is somewhat different, making good decisions is difficult. Making multiple decisions of this sort on a daily basis can be very stressful.

Understanding the pressures your physician experiences may help you see your physician's response to you not as personal but as a function of the practice of medicine. It's also very important to remember that despite these pressures, most physicians are interested in your concerns and dissatisfactions.

What Patients Bring to the Relationship

It also helps to know how the peculiarities of the patient role can shape your dealings with your doctor. Having a physical illness often makes people feel quite vulnerable and less self-sufficient than usual. These two factors together often make patients regress or act more child-like. The doctor then gets placed in the role of parent. This means that any difficulties that existed between you and your parents may show up in your relationship with your doctor. Feelings of emotional deprivation, intrusion, authority conflicts, and so on, may be re-created with your doctor. The limitations of the doctor—little time, the need for emotional distance, and the pressures of making an accurate diagnosis and treatment plan quickly—create fertile ground for these old conflicts to be reenacted. Typically, neither participant is fully aware of the role he or she is playing.

There is a way out of this situation. Think of your specific complaints about your physician. Then ask yourself if any of these complaints are similar to the ones you had or have with your parents. If they are similar in any way, ask yourself whether your expectations of your doctor are too high. Can your doctor realistically be expected to fulfill these expectations given the limitations of the physician role? Has your doctor actually done something to deserve your dissatisfaction? Most often there is a complex combination of these factors. For example, your doctor may have actually done something that made you angry—say, cut you off and left the room before you had finished talking about your concerns—*and* the thing your doctor did was reminiscent of something your parents typically did, such as saying, "Don't talk back to me!" every time you tried to ask a question, raise a problem with their decision, or stage a protest. If you can tease out what your doctor specifically did and view it as an isolated incident rather than a permanent condition, it may be less disturbing to you. It may also be easier to discuss the specific behavior with your doctor. Even if the issue that troubles you has happened repeatedly, identifying the behavior or interaction pattern that is bothersome and keeping yourself from thinking that your doctor's behavior is as unchangeable as the behavior of your parents may help the problem become more manageable. Maryanne, a thirty-two-year-old patient who has had sporadic problems with her asthma since childhood, recounted her experience:

> "Four out of the six times I saw my new doctor, we were interrupted by his nurse telling him he had a call. It always seemed to happen just as he was asking me if I had any concerns. He would leave, and when he came back into the room we never quite got back to my problem. He would do a quick exam, make recommendations, and then leave. I found myself feeling very hurt and disappointed when I thought about him. He was so nice during the first appointment and spent so much time talking to me that I thought we could really work well together to solve the problems raised by my asthma. After the interruptions, I felt like I had to manage on my own. When I was talking to my counselor about it, I started to recall my mother's response to my problems when I was a child.
>
> "I never felt like my mother gave me enough attention. My parents were divorced, and my brother and I lived with my mother most of the time. It seemed like she was so caught up in

her other concerns she didn't have the time or energy to pay attention to me. My brother had lots of behavior problems, so he ended up getting the lion's share of my mother's concern. On the few occasions when something was bothering me enough to trouble her with the issue, she would offer me quick reassurance rather than help me solve the problem. The discussions were always interrupted by my brother's aggressive or dangerous behavior, and my mother would run off and attend to him.

"I realized that my doctor's actions were bringing up old, painful issues for me. With my therapist's help, I was able to separate the problems with my doctor from the problems with my mother. I was able to identify two specific problems I had with my doctor: (1) There seemed to be too many interruptions, and (2) we were never able to discuss my problem to my satisfaction. Once I did this, it was easier for me to develop a plan to talk to my doctor. The interruptions may have been a coincidence, or it may be his style to take calls while with patients. I decided I could ask about this and find out if this behavior was unlikely to happen again or if he was willing to make changes. I also decided that an occasional interruption was understandable and tolerable as long as we were able to continue our discussion when he returned. If, after talking with my doctor, it seemed that the problem could not be changed, I would consider finding a different doctor."

Attitudes toward the Practice of Medicine

Another factor that may pose a problem in the doctor–patient relationship is the attitudes about the physician and medicine that you hold. Some people view medicine and physicians with such extreme mistrust that they see a physician only when their condition is so serious that they have no other choice. This mistrust can lead to conflict because the patient may resist following through with the physician's recommendations. Other people view physicians as miracle workers and expect them to do wondrous things. This too can be problematic because there is no actual cure for asthma—only treatment and management strategies. Anyone placed on that high a pedestal is bound to fall someday. Of course, many patients fall somewhere in between these extreme attitudes. Whatever your attitude, it's helpful to be aware of it so that you can keep it from interfering with your care.

Are My Doctor and I Well Matched?

The personalities of the doctor and the patient, and how well they match, can impact the degree of satisfaction both of the participants feel in the relationship. Sheila's experience is a good example:

❦ "I know my doctor is competent. I had done my homework and found someone with great training and an excellent reputation. 'So, why don't I like him? Why do I dread seeing him?' I would ask myself after each appointment. I wanted someone with a warm bedside manner, someone in whom I could confide and ask difficult questions. Dr. James was just too clinical. I felt I was just another case to him. He also talked so fast I just couldn't seem to keep up or slow him down. By accident one day, I saw his partner instead and discovered she was just the type of physician I wanted. Her casual way of speaking, receptivity to my questions, and caring manner were just right for me. I realized that I wanted her to be my doctor, but I felt it would be very awkward to switch. I really worried about hurting my doctor's feelings and didn't want to confront him. I found that I was avoiding making appointments even when I needed them, because I dreaded his clinical treatment of me. At that point I decided that my health was at stake and that it was important to talk with him. Although it was awkward, he was understanding about the fact that different people like different traits in their doctor. After talking it over with him, I switched my care to his partner. I have been much happier since."

Look through this checklist and ask yourself whether any of these issues impact your relationship with your doctor.

__ My doctor is too emotionally distant and lacks warmth.

__ My doctor is too familiar. I prefer someone with a more professional and distant approach.

__ My doctor talks too fast. I have a hard time following him.

__ My doctor speaks so slowly that I believe he thinks I don't understand.

__ My doctor uses such simple, basic language that I think she thinks I am an imbecile.

__ My doctor uses such complicated terms when she explains things that I can't follow her.

__ My doctor is too controlling. He wants to believe his word is law.

__ My doctor is so flexible that I feel as if I have to make major decisions about my health care, about which I have no information or training.

__ My doctor floods me with too much information. I have a hard time taking it all in.

__ My doctor gives me so little information about my disease process and medications. I feel I'm always in the dark.

__ My doctor has such a relaxed, casual manner that I think she doesn't take anything seriously.

__ My doctor has such a rigid, professional, efficient demeanor that I feel I have to act similarly. It seems there's no room for my feelings.

__ My doctor always seems to minimize my concerns.

__ My doctor takes my concerns so seriously that he enumerates all of the diseases my symptoms could signify, sending me into a panic.

Sometimes these differences can be overlooked if they don't interfere with your care. When they do seem to impact your care, however, talking about them may help. Bringing the issue into the open, so that both of you are more aware of the differences, is a good start. Sometimes one of you can make some adjustments so that the differences don't interfere with your relationship or care. Or it may be that the differences are so great that changing physicians is a good option to consider.

Practical Concerns

Some patients complain that while they get along well with and trust their physicians, other factors cause some resentment or anger. Complaints about practical concerns most often center on (1) money and payment arrangements, (2) accessibility of the physician in urgent situations, and (3) length of time spent waiting for the doctor before each appointment.

Money

Some patients feel their doctor's charges are excessive or out of the range charged by other doctors in their area. At times, the payment arrangement is financially unfeasible or at least difficult for patients. Most often, this happens when patients are asked to pay for the appointment on the same day rather than pay for the balance after their insurance company has been billed. Some patients need to pay over time. The flexibility of the physician around these issues can be very important to patients.

Availability

Patients like to feel that they can get an appointment in a timely manner—even if it is for a routine checkup. Patients often feel better about their physician if evening or weekend hours are available, and they do not have to take time off work. A second part of the availability complaint is how promptly and kindly a physician returns phone calls. Patients tend to feel happier with physicians who return their calls quickly, and who do not seem to resent spending time talking with patients who have a legitimate reason for calling.

Wait before an Appointment

Patients like to be seen promptly once they arrive at the doctor's office. Most are willing to make some allowances about this, but if they are kept waiting too often or too long, dissatisfaction increases.

If any of these issues interfere with your relationship with your doctor, it is a good idea to discuss them with him or her. It may be that your doctor does not recognize the problem and will want to make some changes. Sometimes other arrangements can be made to fit your needs.

The Changing Roles of Doctor and Patient

In the last ten or fifteen years, patients have been encouraged to be informed consumers of health care. This means that patients are generally encouraged to know more about their illness and to be active participants with their physicians in health care decisions. In part, this change was ushered in by more educated consumers and the legal notion of "informed consent." This is a dramatic departure from the medicine practiced of old, in which physicians made decisions and patients followed (or were expected to follow) that advice.

Doctors and patients differ in the extent to which they wish to adopt these new roles. Approaching this issue from divergent viewpoints can cause a great deal of friction in the relationship. Bertha, a sixty-five-year-old patient, complained of this problem:

&> "I really like my doctor for the most part. The difficulty we had at first was that he wanted me to think carefully about the choices he presented me and make my own decision. I wanted him to tell me what to do—that's what I was used to. Once I began talking with him about what I wanted, he shifted his style somewhat. Now he tells me the choices and then gives me his recommendation and reasons for making that choice. All I have to say is, 'It sounds good to me.' Since our little talk, I feel much more comfortable with him. I don't feel so overwhelmed, like so much is expected of me."

Andrea had opposite concerns.

&> "From the moment my asthma was diagnosed, I began to read about the disease and various treatment strategies. I really delved into it, even reading articles from all the latest professional journals. All my reading led me to ask all kinds of questions of my doctor. I wasn't doubting his judgment; I just wanted an open discussion. I also wanted to have a part in major treatment decisions. He didn't take too kindly to this. He seemed to view my questions as a threatening interference. I felt as if he viewed me as a pushy troublemaker. I started to view him as arrogant and insecure. Appointments were painful. I was considering switching doctors and ended up telling him why. He was very concerned about his behavior, apologized, and things have been one hundred percent better since then. He understands I am not questioning his judgment, and I understand that when he tells me what he thinks, it is his recommendation and not an order."

Both of these patients achieved satisfactory results after talking with their doctors. This is not the experience of all patients. Talking is a good first step, but if neither party is really willing to change his or her approach, switching physicians may be the solution.

WHAT TO DO IF YOU ARE DISSATISFIED WITH YOUR DOCTOR

If you feel your doctor is competent but you're dissatisfied with some aspect of your treatment, the best first step is to discuss it. This can be very difficult. Most patients have a hard enough time asking the questions they want to ask. Actually confronting their doctor is much more difficult. Most patients cite intimidation, emotional distance, the doctor's busy schedule, and fears of being seen as stupid as reasons for not questioning or confronting their doctor. Here are some suggestions for how to proceed and tips to make the process easier.

Prepare for the Discussion

The first part of the preparation should be convincing yourself that the discussion is important. Remind yourself of all the reasons why you are unhappy, and make a list. Also list ways this dissatisfaction has interfered with your treatment. Generally, patients who are happy with their care are more likely to follow the doctor's recommendations and are more reliable in keeping appointments and therefore receive better care.

After deciding that it's important, decide how to put your dissatisfaction into words and attempt to come up with a specific example or incident to help describe the situation to your doctor. Avoid accusations or personality attacks. You're much more likely to get a positive response (rather than a defensive one) if you say, "I feel like you don't take my wishes and opinions into account" rather than "You're so arrogant! You always have to have it your way." Concrete examples will help your doctor see your point.

It's also helpful to decide what you want out of the discussion. Do you want an apology? Do you want to come to a compromise or better understanding of the problem? Do you want your doctor to make major changes or minor changes? Are your expectations realistic?

Put Your Plan into Action

When you bring up your concern with your doctor, ask about his or her preference for the timing of the talk. This approach often makes the physician more receptive and makes it possible for the physician to schedule time on a different day if he or she is pressed for time or just having a bad day. Many patients have success with saying, "Dr. _____, there is something that is troubling me about [our interaction, my care, etc.] that I would like to discuss with you. Is today a good day, or should I schedule another time with you?"

Michelle, the patient described at the beginning of this chapter, prepared the following list for her appointment:

Complaints about Dr. Brown:
1) He doesn't listen to me or my worries.

Possible approaches and examples:
"When I told you I was concerned about the effects of prednisone, you said, 'There is nothing to worry about,' instead of asking about my concerns and going over the risks and benefits. If we had done that, we could have decided together if it was right for me to continue on such high doses."

2) He doesn't help with strategies in dealing with dilemmas I face in managing my asthma.

"When I tried to talk with you about the difficulty of taking my medication on time with my changing shift work and erratic sleep schedule, you said, 'Just get an alarm to wake yourself up.' You did not seem to understand that that would mean waking 1 hour after I finally got to sleep."

3) He is so rushed, he doesn't seem to care.

"You never ask me if I have any questions; you just rush out of the room. I end up feeling like I am not important to you or that I am far less important than all of the people you are rushing out the door to see."

What I want out of the discussion:

1) I want Dr. Brown to be more sensitive to my need to be heard and to give me some time at either the beginning or the end of the appointment to ask questions. This is also likely to make me feel more important.

2) I would like Dr. Brown to actually help me come up with realistic strategies to manage my asthma and to fully understand the dilemmas I face.

Unrealistic expectations I have:

It is unlikely that Dr. Brown can make me feel as cared about or as important as I want to feel. That is something I am going to need to work on.

Plan:

Talk with him (or at least schedule a time to talk at my next appointment: Wednesday, March 2, at 2:00). No chickening out!

As she described earlier, Michelle was successful in her attempt to rectify her problems with her doctor. But if talking doesn't change things for you, and you are still dissatisfied, you need to decide whether you can overlook the problems or it's time to look for another physician.

If you decide to keep working with your doctor, the following tactics may help to improve your relationship. These ideas are, in fact, good guidelines for patients with any type of relationship with their doctor.

Strategies for Achieving (or Keeping) a Good Working Relationship with Your Doctor

- Keep a running list of questions you want to ask your doctor and then *ask them*. Do not be put off by the doctor's brusque manner.
- Bring up the fact that you have a number of questions at the beginning of the appointment. Then your physician will be prepared to spend the necessary amount of time with you.
- If you don't understand something, say so. Your doctor will appreciate your questions and is not likely to view you as stupid.
- Take notes while your doctor is giving you instructions. Research suggests that patients remember less than sixty percent of what their physician tells them.
- If your doctor is giving you "orders" that you know you *will not* or *cannot* follow, say so, and explain why. The two of you can then devise an alternate strategy.
- Strive to establish a relationship with your doctor that makes it feel as if the two of you are a team battling your asthma.
- If your doctor does something that makes you unhappy, discuss it as soon as possible after the episode. This will help "clear the air" promptly so that there is no disruption in your care.
- Try to avoid being overdemanding. This attitude proves difficult for most physicians to handle.

Remember, you and your doctor are on the same team, working toward the same goal: helping you live well with asthma. Make the most of the relationship.

ᴥ Appendix

You've read this book and learned ways to live better with your asthma. But don't sit back and relax! There are many resources still available to help you understand asthma and live better with it. Listed below are books, organizations, on-line resources, and activities all intended to help you. Contact the ones that interest you the most. Coping with asthma provides you with new opportunities, to live the way you choose rather than be ruled by an illness.

BOOKS

The Asthma Self-Help Book by Paul J. Hannaway
> This is a useful book for individuals who are just learning about asthma. It defines asthma and describes asthma triggers and treatment methods. There are also informative chapters on environmental controls, air pollution, allergy injections, and childhood asthma.

Asthma: A Complete Guide to Self-Management of Asthma and Allergies for Patients and Their Families by Alan M. Weinstein, MD
> A readable guide to the medical aspects of asthma and how you can help manage it.

Asthma: Stop Suffering, Start Living by M. Eric Gershwin and E.L. Klingelhofer

> This is another basic book about asthma. It describes the disease and typical treatment methods. Some attention is given to self-care.

What You Can Do About Asthma by Nathaniel Altman

> This book describes the disease process as well as many management techniques including environmental management, diet, exercise, and complementary therapies.

A Parent's Guide to Asthma by Nancy Sander

> This book, written by the parent of an asthmatic child, is a very helpful guide for parents. It describes the disease, typical treatments, and gives helpful ideas to parents of asthmatic children.

Children with Asthma: A Manual for Parents by Thomas Plaut

> This is a helpful guide for parents of children with asthma. It addresses many of the concerns and decisions parents have to confront.

Asthma and Exercise by Nancy Hogshed and Gerald S. Couzens

> This book is written by an Olympic gold medalist and explains the helpfulness of exercise for those who have asthma. If you still don't believe that exercise is important, read this book. If you do believe that exercise is important, read this book.

Breathing Disorders: Your Complete Exercise Guide by Neil F. Gordon

> This is another very helpful book on exercise for those with asthma or other breathing disorders.

NEWSLETTERS

LUNG LINE Letter by National Jewish Medical and Research Center

> National Jewish publishes pamphlets, resource lists, and this newsletter on many respiratory and immunological diseases.

MA Report by Allergy & Asthmatic Network/Mothers of Asthmatics
> A monthly newsletter written for people such as parents, doctors, and teachers to help them understand better the needs of children with asthma.

ORGANIZATIONS

National Jewish Medical and Research Center

Not only one of the world's leading asthma treatment centers, National Jewish is an educational resource for any asthma topic. You can call Lung Line and speak with experienced nurses about any aspect of asthma and its treatment. National Jewish also publishes all kinds of material which you can also obtain through Lung Line. To talk with a nurse, call **1-800-222-LUNG** or in Colorado call **303-355-LUNG**.

Allergy & Asthma Network/Mothers of Asthmatics

This organization educates parents, doctors, and teachers about the special needs of children with asthma. Founded by the mother of a child with severe asthma, it publishes a monthly newsletter, pamphlets, and resource lists about pediatric asthma. You can contact this support organization by calling **1-800-878-4403**.

Asthma & Allergy Foundation of America

A foundation intended to educate people about asthma and allergies. It sponsors conferences and training programs and produces publications and audio-visual material. You can contact the foundation by calling **1-800-7-ASTHMA**.

American Lung Association

A nationwide organization with chapters throughout the United States, this association develops information about asthma and many other varieties of lung diseases. It also sponsors publicity events to increase the publics awareness of lung disorders. Call **1-800-LUNG-USA** to contact the national office or look up your local chapter in the phonebook.

Asthma Society of Canada

This society is the only one in Canada devoted solely to asthma. It is a volunteer organization that funds research, runs public education campaigns, publishes a quarterly newsletter, organizes support groups, and administers summer camps for children with asthma. The Asthma Infoline at 1-800-787-3880 can provide you with medical information about asthma (but only if you live in or are visiting Canada). You can contact the Asthma Society of Canada by calling 1-416-787-4050.

Canadian Lung Association

This volunteer association strives to educate the public about a wide range of lung disorders including asthma. Quite striking is its focus upon prevention of lung disease through programs such as promoting smoke-free air in the workplace and other public areas. You can contact the Canadian Lung Association by calling 1-613-747-6776 but it might make more sense for you to call your provincial lung association (there is one for each province and one for the North West Territories) since most of the program services are done at the provincial or municipal level.

ON-LINE RESOURCES

There are thousands of Internet websites that address some aspect of asthma. Unfortunately, it will take you hours to view even a fraction of them and because the Internet is unregulated there is a lot of inaccurate information and unsubstantiated claims. Anyone can develop a website and you can never be sure about their agenda or the validity of their presentation. For example, several websites assert that their products will cure asthma. If you believe that claim, go back and re-read Chapter 1; asthma can be managed but not cured. So beware of what you read! View the Internet as an opportunity to get ideas which you can then discuss with your doctor. By reviewing the information together you foster a collaborative relationship with your physician even if you both agree that the claims are nonsense.

Probably the easiest way to get started on the Internet is by using one of the many search engines that identify different websites after you input one or more keywords. America Online has Netfind that you can access as soon as you request the Internet. Other commercial search engines include **Excite! (www.excite.com), Yahoo! (www.yahoo.com),** and **Alta Vista (www.altavista.com)**. Just type asthma or other, more specific, keywords and you will be presented with brief descriptions of a long list of websites. Then, click on the website which interests you to access it directly.

If you don't want to go through the trouble of surveying all the different websites, Patricia Wrean is a person with asthma who maintains her own asthma and allergy World Wide Web resources page **(www.cco.caltech.edu~wrean/resources.html)**. She lists several sites, some described below, and you can access them directly by just clicking on their name. A less comprehensive asthma and allergy resource website focusing on children also includes links to general information, frequently asked questions, and book reviews **(www.cs.unc.edu~kuptas/FAQ.html)**.

Here are some websites to help you get started. You can find all kinds of strange things on the Internet so these websites were partly chosen because they present more mainstream, widely-accepted medical information.

National Jewish Medical and Research Center (www.njc.org)

This nationally known leader in asthma treatment and research presents a lot of information about the hospital and its physicians. Probably most useful are the topics on their Med Facts page. In the past, National Jewish would send you information after you called their Lung Line. Now, you can view and print immediately any or all their Med Facts papers. A wonderful resource on topics ranging from peak-flow metering to paradoxical vocal cord dysfunction.

Children's Medical Center of the University of Virginia: Asthma Tutorial (www.galen.med.virginia.edu~smb4v/tutorials/asthma)

This is a wonderful website that uses the Internet's multimedia capabilities to illustrate the diagnosis and treatment of asthma. Film and sound clips make this site an entertaining way to learn about asthma. Be patient since the movie and sound bites take a little while to download but it's worth the wait. Although the site focuses on children with asthma, the information readily applies to adults.

Global Initiative for Asthma (www.ginasthma.com)

This world-wide project attempts to increase people's awareness of asthma, identify the reasons why more and more people are suffering from asthma, and improve medical management thereby decreasing asthma deaths. It is a collaborative project between the National Institute of Health's National Heart, Lung, and Blood Institute and the World Health Organization so the long list of international clinicians and researchers is impressive. Most helpful to you will be the various guides to asthma management that you can either view directly or download onto your computer and then look at off-line.

National Heart, Lung, and Blood Institute (www.nhlbi.nih.gov/nhlbi/nhlbi.htm)

This is the NHLBI website and a major funding source for asthma research. You might as well see where your tax dollars are going, and particularly interesting are the Requests for Applications (RFAs), Requests for Proposals (RFPs), and Program Announcements (PAs). Review these initiatives and you can glimpse at new, promising avenues of asthma research which may affect treatment in the years ahead. Yes, the reading can be difficult because of the medical terminology, but try it anyway. You will be surprised how much you can still understand!

CenterWatch (www.centerwatch.com)

This website does not focus solely on asthma but rather lists all kinds of medications currently undergoing clinical trials. This research is primarily required by the Food and Drug Administration before approving a medication for general use and so the pharmaceutical company is paying for it. The website is useful because you can see what advances are being made in the drug treatment of asthma. Also, because the research is listed by state, you can see where and who is doing investigations near you.

American Lung Association (www.lungusa.org)

The website of the American Lung Association has a lot of educational information but the greatest service is that it will e-mail you two electronic newsletters. Just fill in your e-mail address and you will receive automatically both a monthly and a weekly update on asthma research and news. What a great way to keep track of current events! Also, if you are a teenager with asthma, the American Lung Association arranges a weekly chat room for teens with asthma. You can "talk" with others who have asthma and may discover new ways to live better with it.

European Federation of Asthma and Allergy Associations (www.efanet.org)

One of the wonderful things about the Internet is that space really doesn't matter. You can roam around the globe right from your living room. So don't limit your resources to the United States. This website provides a glimpse at European approaches to asthma and most interesting are the EFA Newsletters and the latest European news. Find out how Denmark recommends managing asthma in children! Will Finland halt the increases in asthma by the year 2004? Get some ideas from Europe particularly since new medical treatments are usually approved for use in Europe years before you can find them in the United States.

The American Academy of Allergy, Asthma, & Immunology Website (www.aaaai.org)

This web page describes the Academy, provides some educational information about these illnesses, answers frequently asked questions, provides a resource list, and maintains a list of specialists.

The American College of Allergy, Asthma, & Immunology Online (www.allergy.ncg.edu)

Another website providing educational information about asthma.

ACTIVITIES

So, you don't want to go too far from home because you might have an asthma attack. Or only your doctor understands your asthma and no one in another city will know how to treat you. Or your son must stay home for the summer because all that physical activity at camp will cause breathing problems. Well, if you still have these improbable and unrealistic fears even after trying to unlearn them (see Chapter 3), you can still get away from home. How about a nice cruise to Mexico, Bermuda, or the Caribbean? Several national and local organizations sponsor cruises for people suffering from respiratory problems. The ships are staffed with pulmonology doctors and nurses and are equipped with specialized medical equipment. Not only can you enjoy the ship, the ports-of-call, and being away from home, but there are frequently classes on all kinds of topics such as stress reduction, breathing exercises, and coping skills. You can choose which sessions interest you or you can attend none of them, just enjoy the cruise with the security of knowing that there is an asthma specialist on board. For many people fearful of leaving their hometown because of asthma, such cruises can give them the confidence that they can safely leave home. After having a great time on a cruise, they become a little more adventuresome, going on trips without needing to be tied to their hometown doctor. It's a liberating feeling knowing that you can leave home without fear, worry, and dread. So talk with your doctor, call a local hospital, or contact one of the national organizations listed above and discuss with them cruises or other recreational events staffed especially for people with asthma.

Summertime can be hard for children with asthma. Other kids can run, play, and swim without thinking about their breathing. Unfortunately, that is not always the case with asthmatic children. If the child isn't worried about asthma, a parent certainly is. Yet physical activities are important to children of all ages. It is a primary means by which they develop self-confidence and self-esteem. It also allows them to feel like they are one of the gang. Asthma camps are one place that children can do the physical activities they need and love while being in a safe setting with medical professionals. Generally, children with mild asthma can attend just about any summer camp. But children with moderate, severe, or difficult-to-control asthma can benefit from these specialized summer camps. Asthma camps are also helpful when either the children or their parents are very worried and frightened about asthma attacks; the medical supervision available at such camps decreases such fears. Except for the medical staff, asthma summer camps are quite similar to any other camp. For example, the American Lung Association of Colorado offers Champ Camp at Snow Mountain Ranch in Winter Park, high in the Rocky Mountains. So, not only do the children learn to have fun despite their asthma, they learn that they can do physical activities even at high altitudes; an important lesson if you live in Colorado. During this week in the summer, children ages 7 to 14 participate in the usual menu of camp activities such as hiking, swimming, wilderness skills, arts and crafts, and archery. In addition, there are daily asthma education meetings that teach the children how to better control their asthma by themselves. The medical volunteers, many of whom are members of the Colorado Allergy Society, provide 24-hour medical supervision at the camp. What an excellent way for a child to learn that he is not so different from his peers and that asthma is simply a problem to be solved rather than the primary focus of his life! For children at this age, peer acceptance is so important and opportunities like Camp Champ allow them to feel no different from others and able to lead a normal life with asthma. Many organizations run asthma camps. However, the local chapters of the American Lung Association probably operate the majority of them in the United States and this is a good place to start to obtain further information about them. In fact, the American Lung Association's website **(www.lungusa.org)** describes the camps, making it even easier to find out about them. If you want a Canadian camp, contact the Asthma Society of Canada for information about their camps for asthmatic children.

Dear Health Care Professional,

If you are a medical care provider or psychotherapist treating patients with moderate to severe asthma, you have probably seen first-hand the psychological difficulties that can accompany this disease.

Even the best-informed individuals may be taken off guard by the impact that asthma can have on their emotional and family life. Ask your patients if they have ever heard: "You have asthma? But you don't look sick." How have they handled such comments from well-meaning, but uninformed, friends and family? Have they suffered social embarrassment, or emotional, social, sexual, or occupational difficulties because of their asthma? Are they angry or depressed? Are any of these problems interfering with effective medical management?

This book offers a lifeline to asthma patients attempting to understand and cope with the psychological ramifications of their illness and its treatment. From embarrassment about the use of medications, to anxiety, body image problems, and problems in family functioning, its pages are packed with real-life stories of commonly encountered problems and step-by-step strategies for solving them. Distilling knowledge gleaned from our longtime association with the National Jewish Medical and Research Center, one of the premier centers for the treatment of asthma, our aim is to help patients:

- Identify and break free of faulty beliefs about asthma
- Cope with the emotional aftermath of diagnosis
- Work through psychological barriers to medication use
- Collaborate with family members to solve asthma-related problems
- Manage illness-related occupational problems
- Maintain a healthy social life (and sex life) with asthma
- Establish more productive relationships with physicians

If this book belongs to a colleague or patient, and you are interested in examining it in greater detail, the publisher is making a limited number of examination copies available to health care providers. Call the Guilford Press toll-free at 800-365-7006 to receive your copy which may be examined for 30 days with no obligation to purchase. Please also see the following two pages, which describe two methods for making this resource easily available to your patients.

Michael R. Freedman
Samuel J. Rosenberg
Cynthia L. Divino

PRIORITY ORDER FORM

Send to: **Guilford Publications, Inc., Dept. 4F**
72 Spring Street, New York, NY 10012

CALL TOLL-FREE 800-365-7006
Mon.-Fri., 9 am–5 pm EST
or Fax 212-966-6708

(Be sure to tell the representative you are ordering from our Priority Order form.)

NAME

ADDRESS

CITY   STATE   ZIP

DAYTIME PHONE NO.
(   )

Method of Payment

☐ Check or Money Order Enclosed

Please Bill My: ☐ Visa ☐ MasterCard   ☐ American Express

ACCT. #

☐☐☐☐   ☐☐☐☐   ☐☐☐☐   ☐☐☐☐

Expiration Date: MONTH ☐☐   YEAR ☐☐

SIGNATURE
(Required on Credit Card Orders)

Name of recommending professional:

Please Ship:

Qty.		Cat. #	Amount
1	Living Well with Asthma	0051	$14.95
*shipping Priority Mail — 1 to 2 week delivery		Shipping*	$3.50
		NY and PA add sales tax; Canada add G.S.T.	
		TOTAL	

PRIORITY ORDER
For office use only
**Note: Operator—set up as account
type IT—Mail <u>No</u>—Rush Order
SHIP VIA FC**

Quantity Discounts and a Special Service for Recommending
Living Well with Asthma

To the Health Care Professional:

Here are two convenient methods for ordering *Living Well with Asthma*.

❶ QUALITY DISCOUNTS

For multiple copies of *Living Well with Asthma*, calculate the following discount rates against the list price to get the unit discount price. Then simply multiply the discount price times the quantity you are ordering. Add 5% of your total order for shipping.

QUANTITY	LIST PRICE	DISCOUNT	PRICE PER BOOK
1 book	$14.95	—	$14.95
2-12 books		20% off list price	$11.95
13-24 books		30% off list price	$10.45
25+		33% off list price	$9.85

To order, please call toll-free 800-365-7006

❷ PRIORITY ORDER FORMS

Or, when recommending the book, you may have individuals order directly from Guilford—simply photocopy the Priority Order Form on the next page. Priority Order Forms are given immediate attention.

We also assure confidentiality. Customers who use these order forms will be excluded from the Guilford Mailing list and will receive no further correspondence.

Index